GW01091303

NEW
CONCEPTIONS

NEW CONCEPTIONS

A Consumer's Guide to the Newest Infertility Treatments, Including In Vitro Fertilization, Artificial Insemination, and Surrogate Motherhood

By LORI B. ANDREWS, J.D.

ST. MARTIN'S PRESS • NEW YORK

NEW CONCEPTIONS. Copyright © 1984 by Lori B. Andrews. All rights reserved. Printed in the United States of America. No part of this book may be used or reproduced in any manner whatsoever without written permission except in the case of brief quotations embodied in critical articles or reviews. For information, address St. Martin's Press, 175 Fifth Avenue, New York, N.Y. 10010.

Library of Congress Cataloging in Publication Data

Andrews, Lori B., 1952–
  New conceptions.

  Includes index.
  1. Conception. 2. Infertility—Treatment. 3. Arti-
ficial insemination, Human. 4. Fertilization in vitro,
Human. 5. Surrogate mothers. I. Title.
RG133.A53 1984   618.1'78   83-21202
ISBN 0-312-56610-7

Design by Laura Hammond

First Edition

10 9 8 7 6 5 4 3 2 1

To my bright, beautiful and gutsy mother who,
in a variety of realms,
has helped those around her
conceive the inconceivable.

❦ CONTENTS

xii •

❦ FOREWORD

Old-Fashioned Notions and New Conceptions

by Kenneth J. Ryan, M.D.
Professor and Chairman, Department of Obstetrics and
Gynecology, Harvard Medical School
and Brigham & Women's Hospital, Boston, Massachusetts

There is a popular impression that advances in medical science and technology have created new moral and legal problems for the individual and for society. This appears to be the case with human reproduction, for in trying to decide whether to use modern technology to create new life by circumventing the "natural" sex act with *in vitro* fertilization, we seem to have few precedents to guide our actions—or so it appears. In truth, the problems with new conceptions are variations on a theme about love, sex, marriage and progeny that are as old as Genesis.

Current lifestyles that once shocked but are now creeping into practice include: planned single parenting out of wedlock, parenting by homosexuals, and using artificial insemination by preference rather than need.

We are brought face-to-face with conflicts about sex and having children that have arisen whenever human inventiveness or the anthropological revelations of a Margaret Mead have challenged conventional Western morality. The only thing really new is that with *in vitro* fertilization we have found a way to unite the human egg and sperm outside the body, a "natural" process our evoluting forebears lost when they left their aquatic habitat to live on land. If one does not believe in evolution, one might want to consider *in vitro* fertilization an unnatural act, but the union of sperm and egg is otherwise the same process whether it occurs inside or outside the body.

Even the current practice of seeking another woman to act as a surrogate for an infertile wife has biblical precedent. The first recorded surrogate mother appears to have been Hagar, who, as recounted in Genesis, bore Ishmael for Abraham and Sarah when the latter could not conceive. This seems to have had Divine blessing but was not without some domestic strife.

Some of the questions on the propriety of using sperm obtained by masturbation for artificial insemination depend on the biblical tale of Onan who failed to fulfill Levirate law when he dropped his "seed" on the ground and did not achieve a conception for his dead brother's wife. We still do not know whether he was punished by God for dropping his seed or for failing to fulfill his obligation to maintain his brother's lineage.

Our "old-fashioned" notions have usually been that children should be born of a marriage and that having both an identifiable mother and father living together is a desirable way to start life. Social practices with and without the help of science have challenged these time-honored notions. Before the sex act was "sanitized" by artificial insemination and *in vitro* fertilization, surrogate parenting by either male or female was encumbered only by moral notions and laws about how sex should be conducted between male and female. Society is faced with the need to separate the ethics and laws on sexuality and marriage from evaluation of the technical means of conception and the human ends desired in creating and rearing a child.

Lori Andrews presents in *New Conceptions* all the human drama and social problems that the desire for children in an age of technology entails. When one looks beneath the veneer of science and law, the problems that emerge are hardly new. While technology can replace the sex act, it can never be a surrogate for the role of love and family in a child's life. We at least have 2,500 years of recorded human experience to help guide us.

❦ PREFACE

In our parents' day, marriage and childbirth were expected, added automatically to a person's life like the shiny beads on a child's add-a-pearl necklace. Now more men and women reflect on these decisions. They postpone marriage, perhaps until they have finished college or graduate school. Some husbands and wives deliberate for years about whether and when they should have a child.

For some of us, when we finally decide that we are ready for a child, we learn that a child is not ready for us. We cannot bear children. Various factors in our health, our lifestyle, and our environment are conspiring against us in our desire to have a child.

In the past generation, there has been an increase in the number of people who meet the medical definition of infertility: they have tried to have a child for a year or more with no success. About 15 percent of all couples are infertile.

At the same time that an increasing number of couples are learning that they are infertile, new developments in medical genetics research are making it possible to pinpoint which fertile couples are at risk for passing on a serious genetic defect to their children. When confronted with this information, some couples are choosing not to bear children so that they will not create a seriously ill child.

Now there is new hope for couples who are infertile or have genetic defects. Some of these developments, such as test-tube babies, sperm banks, and surrogate mothers, you may have read about in the newspapers. Others, such as egg donation, artificial embryonation, and embryo adoption, may be totally new to you. All of these methods constitute the New Conceptions.

This book is designed to serve as a complete handbook for people who have tried to conceive and bear a child in the usual

fashion and have failed—or who are worried about conceiving because of genetic reasons. In Chapter One, the latest alternative
means of procreation, the New Conceptions, are described. Chapter Two details why these alternatives are becoming increasingly
popular—and necessary.

• *HOW TO PICK THE RIGHT TECHNOLOGY FOR YOU*

All problems of infertility and genetic defects have what might be
called a PES factor—a Physical, Emotional, and Social component. The physical component is the defect or problem that causes
the couple not to be able to bear a child. With infertility, there
may be difficulty in pinpointing the problem. All too often, the
diagnosis takes a long time, as your friendly physician tells you to
keep trying or you get passed from office to office among various
fertility "experts." Chapter Three of this book is meant to be a
guide to the diagnosis process. It describes in detail the tests that
can be performed and the treatments and new experimental
therapies that can be used for your particular type of problem.

For those whose physical problem is not infertility but the possibility of transmitting a genetic defect, Chapter Four provides information about what tests can be performed to determine
whether you are a carrier of a particular defect, how likely the
possibility is that you could pass it on to your child, and what types
of problems the defect might cause in your child. This will help
you analyze whether you should take the risk of having a child
with your spouse or, if the defect is serious, attempt to avert the
risk with the help of a sperm donor (if the man is the carrier of the
defect) or an egg donor, embryo donor, or surrogate (if the
woman carries the defective gene or chromosome).

Undergoing the appropriate test, however, is only part of the
infertility or genetic struggle. Often, in their search for the physical problem, doctors will fail to deal with the emotional minefield
of infertility or a genetic defect. The husband or wife will be examined like specimens under a microscope, often with little attention

being paid to the emotional turmoil they feel. The shock and disappointment of being unable to bear a child evokes a massive emotional reaction. Failing to understand these reactions can have devastating effects. The emotional turbulence can both damage the marriage and interfere with treatment.

Because pregnancy is something that affects a couple, their emotional reactions to infertility, genetic defects, and alternative methods of conception must be worked out through close communications between the husband and wife. Chapter Five, based on research involving thousands of couples, explains how other people have resolved anxieties, fears, and frustrations about their conditions and treatment. It also describes how they have handled the social aspects of their childlessness, such as whether to tell friends and relatives about their infertility or genetic problems. For many, unnecessary tears were shed and arguments provoked because the husband or the wife was reluctant to voice a particular concern, such as the husband's fear that his wife would no longer consider him virile because of his infertility or genetic problem or the momentary doubt of the wife facing artificial insemination that perhaps she would not be a good mother after all.

• *UNDERSTANDING THE NEW CONCEPTIONS*

The New Conceptions themselves also have PES factors, which are described in detail in Chapters Six through Nine. The physical factor is the manner in which they work to solve the problem in conception. Sometimes this solution creates emotional difficulties of its own. The husband may be left out when the donor sperm is used; similarly, the wife may feel odd being replaced by a surrogate mother. Even when *in vitro* fertilization is used and the child is genetically related to both members of the couple, they may feel the process is too mechanical or may have trouble preparing themselves for the low success rate.

Each method has a social factor as well, consisting of the reaction by the community, religion, and the law. Since scientific advances have separated procreation from sex, it is now possible for a child to have any combination of up to five parents: an egg donor, sperm donor, a woman who provides a womb for all or part of gestation, and the couple who rear the child. In addition, the actual process of conception may be impossible without the intervention of a physician. As more actors get involved in the drama of pregnancy, religious leaders and society at large react with comments on the morality of this involvement. The law is called in to straighten out the rights and responsibilities of all of the participants in procreation.

The PES factors—the physical, emotional, and social components—of *in vitro* fertilization are covered in Chapter Six. The PES factors of artificial insemination are covered in Chapter Seven, and those of surrogate mothering are covered in Chapter Eight. The PES factors of even more avant-garde means of procreation are detailed in Chapter Nine.

The fanfare associated with conceiving through one of these techniques may make it appear that the actual arrival of a New Conceptions child is anticlimactic. That is far from the truth. Your questions will not stop once the child has arrived. You may wonder whether to tell the child about his or her unique origins. You will probably worry about how to avoid treating the child as extremely fragile in response to the extreme effort you have undertaken in creation. Chapter Ten will guide you through these parenting issues.

In the past four years as I put this book together, I attended medical and scientific conferences and visited infertility clinics, sperm banks, *in vitro* fertilization facilities, surrogate mother programs, and other medical and scientific centers across the United States and abroad. Doctors, nurses, scientists, psychologists, psychiatrists, paraprofessionals, and others generously shared their time with me. Even more impressive, though, were the couples who took me into their lives so that their pain, hope, or knowledge could help others in the quest for a child.

"I always wanted to have a family," says Tina. "I picked a career that I felt I could pursue and still raise children. I postponed childbearing and worked to establish myself so that I'd be in a good enough position to take a long maternity leave and spend time with the baby. My husband and I saved and planned. We've done everything we could to create a dream family in which to raise children. But now those children have been denied us."

This book is for people like Tina—to give them hope and to teach them about the latest means to find the joys of parenting.

New
Conceptions

1 ❦ Introducing the New Conceptions

Linda is thirty-six years old. She has been trying to have a child for five years. "I was poked, prodded, and embarrassed by doctors for three years before I was told last year that a scarring in my fallopian tubes was the cause of the problem," she recalls. "I cried for days, thinking this was all my fault, that I should have married younger than thirty-one if I really wanted a child.

"Now I'm trying to do something about it," Linda continues. "One of the American test-tube baby clinics has turned me down because I'm too old, but another still has my application and I'm hoping it will accept me. If not, I guess I'll have to deal with the idea of a surrogate mother. We're afraid to do that right now because of that case where the surrogate decided to keep the couple's child. I'd be just devastated if that happened to me. Then I will have failed in two different ways to become a mother."

If you are reading this book, you may be going through the same series of crises as Linda. You or your spouse, or maybe both of you, may be among the ten to twenty million Americans who are infertile.

Until recently, the advice to infertile couples was "just keep trying." Keep trying by making love on certain days before your temperature reaches certain levels. Keep trying while he is taking a drug like Clomid or Serophene to enhance his sperm count or she is taking a medicine like Pergonal to increase her fertility. Keep trying through various self-help measures such as his wearing baggy undershorts (so that body heat around the sperm will not cause it to develop abnormally) or her lying quietly for a half hour after lovemaking to ensure that the sperm have a fair shot at making the trek to the egg. Keep trying after painful operations to correct some problem in the reproductive system that he or she may have.

Even with all that trying—on various days, in particular positions, through countless treatments—you still might fail to conceive. Worse yet, you may wonder what ever happened to the joy of sex. The emotional pressures may be too much for even the most loving couple to bear without some ugliness coming out—like the accusation, "It's all your fault," or the desperate fights when one of you seems not to be trying as hard anymore.

• *THE STATISTICS OF INFERTILITY*

The problem of infertility is not new. The Bible is replete with women, like Sarah and Rachel, who were barren. History brings us such tales as well, with an occasional king disposing of his queen if she could not produce an heir. In the past generation, however, there has been an astonishing rise in the infertility rate—the percentage of couples who cannot conceive a child after one year of trying.

William Mosher of the National Center for Health Statistics recently compared two surveys—one taken in 1965, the other in 1976—that are the most recent attempts to access fertility on a national level. He found an 83 percent increase in infertility among married couples in which the wife was between twenty and twenty-four years of age, traditionally a most fertile group. The 1976 survey found that about 10 percent of all married couples were infertile. Now the figure is estimated to be about 15 percent.

"The actual figures for infertility are much higher than that," claims Martin O'Connell, chief of the Fertility Statistics Branch of the Census Bureau. "These surveys label 'infertile' a married woman who has tried to have a child in the past year and failed. But there are many women who are infertile and just don't realize it yet because they haven't tried to have a child.

"Also, by just surveying *married* women, the surveys miss the many women under age thirty who aren't married," adds O'Connell. These unmarried women who postpone childbearing may be at an especially high risk for developing infertility problems.

When the causes of a couple's infertility are investigated, a male problem is found primarily responsible 40 percent of the time, a female problem 40 percent of the time, and a combination 20 percent of the time. A couple may have a problem conceiving a child even if both were fertile earlier in their lives or achieved pregnancies with other partners. Like the growth in primary infertility, there has been an increase in the number of couples with secondary infertility, who successfully give birth to one child and then find that they cannot achieve another pregnancy. For every three couples who are infertile and childless, there are two couples who have become infertile after having children.

The social trend toward postponing childbearing also affects the ability to conceive. Peak fertility for both men and women occurs between the ages of 20 and 25.

In a survey done in June 1981, 3,381,000 American women said they had given birth to a child in the previous twelve months. According to even the most conservative estimates, however, another four million couples tried to get pregnant during that period and could not. These people come from all races, all religions, and all economic and social backgrounds. For virtually all, infertility presents an unparalleled life crisis.

The devastation of infertility would not be so great were it not for another social trend—the decreasing number of babies available for adoption. Widespread use of contraceptives and abortion has led to fewer adoptable children, and more unwed mothers are deciding to keep their children. While in 1971, 13 percent of unwed teenage mothers chose adoption, only 4 percent of those giving birth in 1978 did so. In California today, about 97 percent of the unwed mothers of all ages decide to keep their children and rear them.

• *THE FACES OF INFERTILITY*

Stella and Jim Baer (not their real names) have been trying to have a child since they married thirteen years ago. Stella has gotten pregnant twice, but both times she miscarried very late in the pregnancy.

An outsider would think that the Baers have a charmed life. They are attractive, obviously in love, and enjoy traveling together. Their stunning high-rise apartment overlooks a panoramic skyline. A photo album rests on the cocktail table, with pictures of a European vacation they probably could not have afforded if they had had children.

But the Baers are longing to move on to the next stage of their life. They want to share their love with a child. Their years of trying unsuccessfully to add a new member to their family have chipped away at their self-esteem. They shun social engagements, fearing that their infertility shows and that everyone will think they are defective. They long to get rid of their temperature charts, empty the medicine cabinet, and cancel doctor appointments. They would gladly trade *anything* they own, any experience or opportunity they have had, for the child they so desperately want.

Stella follows the medical developments more closely than even the top infertility specialists. She and Jim will travel to another state if a doctor there has a new approach. She tracks down scholarly scientific articles through a local medical association library. "My biggest fear," remarks Stella, who is now thirty-seven, "is that they will find a cure for my type of problem and that I will be just a little too old for it to do us any good."

• *NEW HOPE FOR INFERTILE COUPLES*

The Baers have tried drugs, surgery, and other medical interventions to help them have a child together through regular intercourse. If you, like them, have tried these approaches and failed, the science of reproductive technology offers stunning new means of achieving parenthood. Medically, they range from extremely simple (artificial insemination) to amazingly complicated (the test-tube baby technology). They all have one thing in common: they require letting a third (and sometimes even fourth or fifth) party into the marriage relationship.

TEST-TUBE BABIES

In some cases, the additional party will be a doctor who performs *in vitro* fertilization (IVF). This is the test-tube baby technique made famous with the birth of Louise Brown in 1978. The doctor will operate on the wife to remove an egg from her ovary, then put it in a shallow dish filled with a special medium and add some of her husband's sperm. If the procedure "takes" and the egg is fertilized, the doctor will act as a "parent," in some senses, for a few days, ensuring that the right amounts of nutrients are in the dish for the embryo to begin to divide. Then he or she will remove the embryo from its temporary resting place in the laboratory and implant it back in the real home, the wife's uterus, so that she may give birth nearly nine months later to a child that is hers and her husband's.

In vitro fertilization is the new reproductive technology that most closely resembles natural childbearing, since the child that is born is genetically 100 percent the couple's. The baby is the result of the merging of the wife's egg and the husband's sperm. In the other new techniques, however, the child may have the genes of only one of the marriage partners or maybe neither.

ARTIFICIAL INSEMINATION

When artificial insemination by donor (AID) is used, the third party who activates the conception is a male donor of sperm. Sperm from a donor is used when sperm from the husband can't be. Perhaps the husband is infertile because of a low sperm count, exposure to a hazardous working environment, or a drug that he is taking for cancer or some other disease. Maybe he had a vasectomy that could not be reversed.

The procedure for artificial insemination by donor is a simple one. When the wife is about to ovulate, she visits a doctor's office. She assumes the position for a pelvic examination and the doctor either uses a syringe to squirt a donor's sperm into her vagina near the cervix or inserts the sperm in the vagina in a diaphragmlike cervical cap that the woman will wear for the following four to six hours.

SURROGATE MOTHERHOOD

For every couple who needs to let a male donor into the relationship to create a child, there is another that needs the aid of a female. A woman's reproductive cycle is extremely complicated. To achieve a pregnancy, an egg must be released from the woman's ovaries, travel down the fallopian tube, be fertilized by sperm, and implant itself in the uterine wall. The infertile woman might call upon another woman's aid for any number of steps in this process.

Already, hundreds of couples have called upon surrogate mothers to help them bear children. A surrogate mother is a woman who agrees to be inseminated with the sperm of a man whose own wife is not capable of conceiving or carrying a child to term. She carries the child for nine months and then, after its birth, signs it over for adoption by the couple.

EGG DONATION

In Italy, a doctor has developed a technique for egg donation in which the microscopic egg of a woman donor is transferred into the wife who cannot produce her own egg or whose own eggs cannot make the trek to the uterus. It is hoped that, once the egg is inside the wife, it will be fertilized by her husband's sperm through natural intercourse and she will give birth to a child nine months later in the usual manner.

ARTIFICIAL EMBRYONATION

Closer to home, in Los Angeles and Chicago, fertility clinics are beginning to offer artificial embryonation (AE), where the donor female provides more than the egg. If the wife is infertile because she does not produce eggs or because her fallopian tubes are damaged, she may still be able to bear a child. With artificial embryonation, the childless husband and wife pay a fee to a fertile woman who agrees to be inseminated with the husband's sperm. Then, four to five days after fertilization, doctors try to flush out the embryo so that it can be implanted in the wife, just as the embryo would be if *in vitro* fertilization had been used.

EMBRYO ADOPTION

If the wife has an ovarian or tubal problem and her husband is sterile as well, a variation of the artificial embryonation procedure, known as embryo adoption (EA), is possible. The volunteer is inseminated not by the husband's sperm but by the sperm of a donor. The embryo is again flushed out after five days and implanted to grow to term in the wife. The embryo has genes from neither member of the couple, even though the wife will bear the child. Both AE and EA are forms of embryo transfer after *in vivo* (in the body) fertilization.

• *THE GENETIC APPLICATIONS OF THE NEW CONCEPTIONS*

The techniques of artificial insemination, egg or embryo transfer, and surrogate mothering offer new hope not only for infertile couples but also for couples wishing to avoid passing on genetic defects. A couple may use artificial insemination by donor rather than risk the husband's passing on a genetic disorder such as Huntington's chorea; they may turn to a surrogate mother if the wife is carrying the gene for hemophilia and does not want to risk having an afflicted son. Many couples' reproductive systems function perfectly, but one or both are afraid they will pass on a genetic defect.

If both members of the couple carry the gene for a recessive disorder, they will both be healthy, but there will be a 25 percent chance that they will have an affected child. Ironically, both of them would be able to have a healthy child if they conceived with someone else.

Such couples have a range of choices that was unavailable as recently as their parents' generation. They could conceive a child together and undergo amniocentesis during the pregnancy to determine whether the child is affected with the genetic disease. If the child is affected, they will then face the heart-wrenching decision of whether or not to undergo an abortion.

As an alternative, couples who are carriers of a recessive genetic defect could turn to the New Conceptions. The wife could undergo artificial insemination with the sperm of a donor who is not a carrier and the husband could conceive a child via the artificial insemination of a surrogate. That way, rather than having one child who is totally theirs genetically (and risks being affected by a serious genetic defect), they will have two healthy children, each genetically related to one of them.

• *COPING WITH THE EMOTIONAL AND PHYSICAL PROBLEMS OF INFERTILITY*

If you are considering using one of the New Conceptions, you must determine whether it is right, both physically and emotionally, for you and your spouse. Often this means that you will both have to come to terms with your feelings about the infertility or genetic problem and the reproductive technology that will be used to alleviate it.

Take the case of Shirley, a fertile woman whose husband's low sperm count made him sterile. Shirley appeared to be the perfect candidate for artificial insemination. But when the artificial insemination was tried, nothing happened. The emotional upheaval between the couple caused Shirley's otherwise perfect ovulatory cycle to be thrown off, and thus there was no egg ready to be fertilized when the donor sperm was introduced into Shirley's reproductive system. Not until the emotional problems were resolved did Shirley's cycle return to normal and she become pregnant.

Since doctors often do not provide emotional counseling, it is important for the husband and wife themselves to analyze their emotional reactions. Some find help through participation in a local chapter of Resolve, a self-help organization for infertile couples.

For many couples, the initial reactions in learning about their infertility or genetic problem are disbelief, then guilt, then anger. Discovering they are infertile may be an ironic blow to a couple who in the past may have been carefully practicing birth control and now learn that it was never necessary. For people with a serious genetic defect, their first shocking realization that they have a problem may come when they give birth to a seriously ill child.

The initial shock causes people to respond, "This can't be happening to me." This disbelief may trigger a type of denial, where they feel the diagnosis is some sort of mistake. Even though they hear it over and over again from many different doctors, they may refuse to face the situation and continue submitting to test after test by doctor after doctor rather than explore the possibility of parenthood via one of the new reproductive technologies.

The second stage—guilt—begins when the spouse with the problem wonders why he or she was apparently singled out for this tragedy. Guilt is particularly pronounced when the individual comes from a large family or has brothers or sisters who conceive frequently or easily.

The partner who cannot bear children may become obsessed with determining whether the problem might have been averted. He or she might wonder if job environment caused the infertility or the genetic defects in his sperm. The man might bemoan the fact that he had a vasectomy after having children with his first wife, without considering the fact that he might marry again and wish to have children with his second wife. A woman may also engage in extensive "what ifs." Like Linda, she may fault herself for not marrying at an earlier age. Or, since having a variety of sexual partners increases the risk of infertility, the man or woman may feel infertility is a punishment for an earlier sexual relationship.

After disbelief and guilt, the person experiences anger. Although it is anger at the situation, it may be expressed through lashing out at the spouse. The person's sensitivity makes it difficult for the spouse to figure out how to act. At times, the spouse with the problem, for example, the wife, may be angry at her husband because she feels he does not understand all she is going through.

At other times, she may lash out because she feels he is trying too hard to understand and is dwelling on the matter so much that it makes her feel like a freak.

Many things can be done to counter these emotional reactions. The first is to stop trying to rewrite your past. Each one of us carries four to ten genetic defects that can affect our offspring with varying degrees of severity. Two out of every one hundred babies have severe birth defects. You are not alone or abnormal if genetic concerns figure in your childbearing calculus.

Likewise, infertility affects at least ten million people in the United States; it is a medical problem, not a moral one. Even if there is something in your past that you would have done differently, there is no way of knowing whether such a difference would have guaranteed fertility. Most likely, it could not have because certain trends affect all men and women, no matter what they do, and many infertility problems result from a combination of causes.

This complicated biological process can be affected in dozens of ways beyond the individual's control. The infertility problem may be physiological—caused by the positioning of a woman's uterus or a man's testicles. It can be environmental—for instance, pollution apparently has caused men's sperm count to drop 30 percent in the past fifty years. Each year, dozens of new factors are implicated in the increase in infertility. A study by Dr. Mona Shengold of Albert Einstein Medical School found that long-distance running by women causes hormonal changes that can lead to infertility. Another study found that male operating room personnel experience decreased fertility and a higher likelihood of their wives' miscarrying, apparently due to contact with anesthetic gases. In such a complicated medical area as this, "what ifs" are particularly misplaced.

There are other reasons why self-blame is inappropriate. "Infertility problems are problems of the couple rather than those of just the man or the woman," comments urologist Dr. Richard Amelar of New York University School of Medicine. Amelar conducts a male infertility practice with his partner, Dr. Lawrence Dubin. "It takes two people to have a baby, but many times this is forgotten in the medical evaluation." The doctor may examine the woman, find an infertility problem, and begin treating it without sufficient study to see whether her husband, too, has something wrong with him. This one-sided test could lead to the woman feeling isolated and blameworthy even when both spouses have a fertility problem.

A particularly striking example of one-sided diagnosis is the case of a man who was born with no testicles. Naturally, he and his wife, were unable to have children. His younger brother, however, volunteered to donate a testicle to him and the transfer was done in a complicated surgery.

The happy man was now sure that he could become an even happier father. After months of trying, however, he and his wife still could not conceive. Finally, his wife was checked and found to have her own problem of infertility. After she was treated with drugs, they were able to have a baby at last.

• *HOW SOCIETY VIEWS THE NEW CONCEPTIONS*

In addition to their physical and emotional components, infertility, genetic defects, and their treatment have wide-ranging social ramifications as well. In 1966, S. J. Kleegman and S. A. Kaufman, in *Infertility in Women,* made the observation that new reproductive technologies are greeted initially with shock and must pass through several stages before they are accepted. "Any change in custom or practice in this emotionally charged area has always elicited a response from established custom and law of horrified negation at first; then negation without horror; then slow and gradual curiosity, study, evaluation, and finally a very slow but steady acceptance," they wrote. Their statement focused on artificial insemination, but the same could be said of *in vitro* fertilization, surrogate parenting, egg donation, artificial embryonation, embryo adoption, and genetic counseling.

Unfortunately, many people are still stuck in the initial stages of shock over the New Conceptions. In their panic, they argue that the new reproductive technologies should not be used because they are unnecessary, selfish, unnatural, and dangerous.

"Though it saddens the life of many infertile couples, infertility is hardly one of our major social problems," asserts University of Chicago biologist and ethicist Leon Kass. The chairman of the British Medical Association's central ethics committee put it even more bluntly: "After all," he declared, "you don't die of infertility."

At a time when overpopulation is rampant and funding for medical research is scarce, some scientists believe that it is irresponsible to pursue research on reproduction technologies. An editorial in the *Journal of the American Medical Association* in 1972 advocated a moratorium on *in vitro* fertilization research, relying in part on Kass' assertion that infertility is not a disease, just a desire to have children. Ethicist Marc Lappé counters that, "when we speak of justification for medical practice, we are talking simply about a universal obligation to relieve suffering. And childlessness is a particularly acute form of such suffering."

Dr. Robert Edwards and Dr. Patrick Steptoe, fathers of *in vitro* fertilization, likewise take issue with the claim that the cure for overpopulation is denying treatment to infertile couples. "Adopting this suggestion," they point out, "would lead to changes in the doctor-patient relationship and could demand that an unfortunate minority be penalized for the sake of the majority."

Even among people who view the infertile couple's goal of becoming parents as a respectable one, there are those who oppose the new methods because of their seeming unnaturalness. According to theologian G. R. Dunstan, "The further the act of insemination is removed, for instance, from the personal union and common life of the donor and recipient of the seed, the further from the human and therefore the more suspect morally the practice would be." Similar criticism has been leveled for turning the marriage bed into a scientific laboratory.

In vitro fertilization practitioner Dr. Howard Jones of Norfolk, Virginia, challenges the idea that the new technologies are unethical manipulations of nature. "Actually, every request of a physician to diagnose and treat disease is a request to manipulate nature," he notes. "If it is ethically acceptable to seek medical care for a reproductive disorder, it is ethically acceptable to seek care which requires *in vitro* fertilization."

The most compelling argument against the New Conceptions is

that they could lead to massive unacceptable changes in society. Widespread availability of amniocentesis and abortion might lead to cutbacks in support to the handicapped and discrimination against such children on the grounds that parents could have chosen not to give birth to an affected child in the first place. Acceptance of the use of egg donors, sperm donors, and surrogate mothers might lead to a couples' attempts to create superkids—for example, by choosing as a donor a famous scientist or musician. In the process, the children will lose the right to be unique as their parents pressure them to pursue the same activities as their successful progenitors.

These are indeed serious concerns. But banning techniques such as genetic counseling, artificial insemination, and *in vitro* fertilization today is not necessary to protect against abuses in the future. The best way to guard against these dangers is for concerned people to make their voices heard about the proper use to which the new technologies are to be put. Decisions that go to the very heart of what it means to be human should not be left to the scientists alone.

"Infertile people perhaps have a clearer sense of the meaning of parenthood than those who come to it with less effort," asserts Chicago infertility counselor Judy Calica. "Because they are stuck in the process of becoming a parent for such a long time, they have given more thought to the meaning of having children." It is this special perspective that couples like you can bring to the societal debate about the benefits and misuses of the new reproductive technologies.

• *HOW RELIGION AND THE LAW VIEW THE NEW CONCEPTIONS*

Your quest to become a parent through the New Conceptions or your attempt to lobby for more widespread availability of these options will have formidable opponents. Two powerful societal institutions—the church and the legal system—have, at various points, attempted to discourage the new reproductive technologies.

Both the Catholic and Orthodox Jewish religions have taken a position against many of these techniques, while the Protestants and Reform Jewish faiths generally approve or condone them.

According to Paul Ramsey, a theologian at Princeton University, the use of a reproductive technology that lets a third party into the marriage relationship via artificial insemination, surrogate mothering, or embryo transfer "puts completely asunder what God joined together." But Episcopalian theologian Joseph Fletcher disagrees. He thinks such a technology can strengthen a marriage. It is not harmful, maintains Fletcher, since parenthood is "a moral relationship with children, not a material or merely physical relationship."

Courts, and legislators, too, have not been entirely supportive of embryo technologies. A few judges have held that artificial insemination by donor constituted adultery and that the resulting child is illegitimate. Surrogate motherhood is banned in a number of states as illegal baby-selling. In some states, doctors decline to perform *in vitro* fertilization because of strict laws designed to protect fetuses.

The New Conceptions all require couples to call on the aid of other people to help them bear children. These people may be physicians, sperm donors, egg donors, or women who will carry the children. In all these situations the legal saga could be entitled "Whose Child Is It Anyway?" since the extra participants have rights and responsibilities of their own toward the child. There are legal problems in determining whether the legal mother is the person who provides the egg, who carries the child, or who raises the child after birth. The father's legal status is also in question.

The laws of artificial insemination, surrogate mothering, *in vitro* fertilization, and other embryo technologies are in flux. That is why it is necessary for a couple considering any of these techniques to pick the approach that is best tailored to them legally as well as medically. Do not be discouraged by the thicket of legal regulation, though. Once you know the law, you can arrange for the procreation process (for example, the embryo adoption or the insemination of the surrogate) to take place in a location with favorable rules on the subject.

Societal thinking has not yet caught up with the new reproductive technologies. As you learn about the physical, emotional, and social components, you can choose the techniques that are best for you and begin to forge the way for their acceptance and availability.

2 ❦ *Hazards to Fertility*

Despite the fact that infertility affects one couple out of six, some infertile couples cannot believe that it is happening to them. When Ken and Janet Robertson (not their real names) could not seem to get pregnant once they tried, it did not dawn on them that they had a fertility problem. They used various excuses to explain why Janet had not gotten pregnant—maybe they had not made love at the right time of month or maybe Janet was arising too soon after lovemaking.

Janet and Ken developed excuses to avoid lovemaking so they would not try and fail. Ken saw a doctor who told him, erroneously, that his boderline sperm count would prevent them from ever having children. Janet went to a psychotherapist who told her that her infertility was due to psychological unwillingness to choose between child and career. They started blaming each other for their barrenness and, feeling that the problem must be with their marriage, spoke to lawyers about a divorce. As a last-ditch effort, though, they vowed to learn enough about reproduction and their own bodies so they would not be leaving any stone unturned.

• *HOW DOES PREGNANCY OCCUR?*

The reproductive process is a stunningly complex one. "As a spectacle it can be compared only with an eclipse of the sun, or the eruption of a volcano," wrote Dr. G. W. Corner in 1942. "If this were a rare event, or if it occurred only in some distant land, our museums and universities would doubtless organize expeditions to witness it, and the newspapers would record its outcome with enthusiasm."

For the woman, the chemicals that orchestrate a pregnancy are the hormones. Each month, a specific hormone, FSH (follicle-stimulating hormone), sends a message to the woman's ovaries to begin maturing an egg in one of the ovarian follicles for ovulation. Midway through the woman's monthly cycle, another hormone, LH (luteinizing hormone), triggers the release of the egg.

If all is well, the woman's fallopian tube that is closest to the ovary releasing the egg will extend and cover up the follicle that contains the egg. When the egg leaves the ovary, it will travel down that tube. The egg will remain fertile for only about twelve hours. Sperm can remain fertile for around forty-eight hours, so even if the couple makes love two days before ovulation, the sperm can linger in the woman's body awaiting the release of an egg.

Various changes occur within the woman to aid in the meeting between egg and sperm. For example, there is a dramatic evolution in the mucus covering the cervix, the entryway to the uterus through which the sperm must pass in their journey from the vagina into the uterus and ultimately to the fallopian tubes. Near the time of ovulation, the woman produces extra estrogen, which increases the amount of mucus and makes it clear, watery, and stretchable. At other times of the month, the mucus resists penetration by the sperm. The increased estrogen changes the mucus so that it can be penetrated more readily by the sperm.

Meanwhile, the follicle from which the egg emerged has begun to produce more hormones—estrogen and progesterone—which cause an accumulation of blood and other nutrients in the uterus. If the egg is fertilized in the tube, it then travels down the fallopian tube and will implant itself in the rich uterine lining and develop into a fetus. If the egg is not fertilized, the uterine lining will be shed (that is, the woman will menstruate) usually fourteen days after ovulation. When the woman's period starts, so too begins a cycle. FSH is again released and the process starts anew.

Any number of things can go wrong in this complicated ritual.

The initial hormones may be weak or missing, so that no message is sent for an egg to ovulate. Or the message may be sent too late, so that an overly ripe, unfertilizable egg is released. Or insufficient hormones may be produced, failing to prepare the uterus for implantation. The woman's abdomen may contain adhesions—a buildup of scar tissue caused, for example, by an appendectomy or an infection, which makes it impossible either for the ovary to release the egg or for the tube to move toward the ovary. The tube itself could be blocked, preventing the meeting of egg and sperm. The cervical mucus could be "hostile," denying the sperm entry. Or the uterine lining could be inhospitable, preventing a fertilized egg from implanting or causing a miscarriage after implantation. Chromosomal or genetic abnormalities in the embryo—introduced either by the man's sperm or the woman's egg—could also cause the embryo to miscarry.

Hormones guide a complicated scenario in the man, too, as he manufactures sperm. While a woman is born with all the eggs she will use in a lifetime, a man's body must continually create sperm. Two hormones, FSH and LH, stimulate the production of sperm in the tubes in a man's testicles. The sperm develops through several stages, assembly-line fashion, over a period of around seventy-two days; it takes an additional three weeks for the mature sperm to travel through the man's ducts. A properly developed sperm has an oval head and a long, thin tail. It can move quickly in a straight line by moving its tail. An improperly developed sperm may have a round head, an elongated head, two heads, or some other deformity or it may move too slowly in a circular motion.

In addition to needing a high-quality sperm, a man, in order to be fertile, needs a considerable quantity of sperm, since 99.9 percent of the sperm that enter the woman during lovemaking never get beyond the vagina for a potential meeting with the egg in a fallopian tube. In addition, there must be a clear pathway for the sperm to travel through during ejaculation. If the man's tubes are blocked, even the healthiest sperm cannot reach the woman's body for a shot at fertilizing an egg.

Sperm development is also sensitive to temperature—sperm will not be produced if the temperature in the testes is over 95 degrees Fahrenheit. (This is why the testes hang away from the body—so they can maintain a lower temperature than the rest of the body). If a man has, say, a viral infection that raises his temperature, his ability to produce sperm will be lessened, and three months after the fever, there may be fewer or less active sperm in his semen.

Although a man with just a few healthy sperm could conceivably initiate a pregnancy, the sperm quality standards for a man to be considered of "normal" fertility are high. When semen is examined under the microscope (in a sperm count), there should be a volume of two to five cubic centimeters, with at least twenty million sperm per cubic centimeter of semen. At least fifty percent of the sperm should have normal shapes and move in the normal, straight manner.

• *NEW CAUSES OF INFERTILITY*

The way we reproduce has remained the same since the dawn of humanity. Since the *process* is the same, what are the culprits that now impede fertility in a growing number of couples?

The new causes of infertility vary widely, but the bulk of them have this in common: an advance in some other area of our lives or society has hampered fertility. Changes occurred and nobody asked about their effect on fertility. For example, new drugs and medical devices were introduced on the market for other uses (such as easing ulcers) without sufficient consideration of their effect on fertility. New chemicals were devised and produced in factories without enough testing of their influence on workers' procreative capabilities. Since the late 1960s, a new lifestyle has evolved, with couples postponing childbearing without sufficient information on how the decision influences their chances in the reproduction gamble.

WHAT'S YOUR FERTILITY QUOTIENT?

The medical definition of infertility is the inability to conceive after a year of unprotected intercourse or the inability to carry a pregnancy to term. However, many people wonder about how fertile they are *before* they make a full year's attempt. Some have a suspicion that they may be infertile; others have no intention of becoming a parent for years but still wonder whether they will be able to.

Although a definitive diagnosis of infertility should be made by a physician after pursuit of the various tests described in this book, a yes answer to any of the following questions indicates that you are at an increased risk of infertility when compared with the average population.

QUESTIONS FOR WOMEN:

Have you had pelvic inflammatory disease?

Have you used an IUD?

Have you had an infection of the reproductive organs after an abortion?

Have you undergone abdominal surgery—for example, for appendicitis?

Are you taking any medications that could be diminishing your fertility?

Do you come in contact with lead or other hazardous substances in your workplace?

Have you undergone chemotherapy or radiation therapy or do you work with such substances?

Have you been treated for a cervical infection by cautery (burning) or cryosurgery (freezing) of the cervical area?

Do you live in a heavily polluted area or one that is frequently sprayed with pesticides?

Did your mother take DES when she was pregnant with you?

Do you use a lubricant during lovemaking that could be destroying sperm?

Have you postponed childbearing until you are in your 30s or 40s?

WHAT'S YOUR FERTILITY QUOTIENT?

QUESTIONS FOR MEN:
Have you had an infection of the reproductive organs, such as venereal disease?

Did you have mumps during puberty?

Have you had a hernia repair or other abdominal surgery during which the vas deferens may have accidentally been severed?

Are you taking any medications (for conditions such as ulcers or high blood pressure) that could be diminishing your fertility?

Do you come into contact with lead or other hazardous substances in your workplace?

Have you undergone chemotherapy or radiation therapy or do you work around radioactive substances?

Do you live in a heavily polluted area or one that is frequently sprayed with pesticides?

Did your mother take DES when she was pregnant with you?

Have you been exposed to Agent Orange?

Are you currently exposed to any reversible threats to fertility such as heating of the testicles due to tight underpants, hot baths, or sitting in the same position for long periods of time (such as while driving a truck)?

Do you use a lubricant during lovemaking that could be destroying sperm?

POLLUTION AND OTHER ENVIRONMENTAL HAZARDS

The modern world is a harsh one, particularly on the development of sperm. Dr. Ralph Dougherty, professor of chemistry at Florida State University in Tallahassee, found that many chemical pollutants were lowering men's sperm counts. While forty years ago less than 5 percent of men tested had sperm counts of less than twenty million per cubic centimeter (the lower limit of normal), 23 percent of the men Dougherty tested in 1979 were in that category. That means that nearly one quarter of Dougherty's sample— college students—would be considered infertile on the basis of their sperm counts.

"The trend is sufficiently dramatic," warns Dougherty, "that it is becoming imperative to find out what the cause is. I'm hoping that the scientific community will rise to the challenge and investigate the relationship of chemicals to infertility."

In addition to general pollution, specific chemicals in the air may be hazardous to your reproductive capabilities. Following the spraying of the herbicide Silvex in Oregon towns, the rate of miscarriages rose so rapidly that the Environmental Protection Agency banned its use in forest areas. But, according to Dougherty, it is still sprayed over flatlands and rice fields, primarily in California and Arkansas.

WORKPLACE HAZARDS

Certain job environments also hamper fertility by lowering a man's sperm count or by causing a woman to menstruate irregularly or by introducing chromosomal abnormalities into the sperm, the egg, or the embryo. Potential fertility hazards abound for workers who deal with lead, pesticides, polystyrene, xylene, some solvents, benzene, and mercury. People in the health care industry may also be at risk, since a certain level of contact with radioactive materials or anesthetic gas also adversely affects fertility.

Often, the fertility risk is uncovered only by chance. In the case of the herbicide dibromochloropropane, explains Dr. Paul W. Brandt-Rauf of the Columbia Presbyterian Medical Center in New York City, "a number of male workers were sitting around talking and they realized that they were all having trouble trying to have children." Tests revealed that the chemical was so hazardous to sperm that it is now no longer produced in the United States.

Even jobs that involve no hazardous materials can decrease fertility. Research has found that sitting too long in one place (some executive desk jobs or driving a truck or cab) raises the temperature in the testes and, thus, impedes sperm production. Stress, including extreme job stress, can throw off a woman's ovulation; scientists speculate that it can lower a man's sperm count as well. Fortunately, unlike the effect of many hazardous substances, these problems can be overcome once recognized by the individual as the cause of his or her infertility.

TREATMENT TECHNOLOGIES

Some fertility problems have been caused, ironically, by doctors treating other maladies. For example, in the mid-1950s doctors prescribed DES (di-ethyl-stilbestrol) to women to prevent miscarriages. Now, though, the daughters of the women who took DES are trying to have their own children and a significantly high number are discovering that they are infertile. It seems that the DES caused some of them to have kinked-up tubes (impeding the meeting of sperm and egg) or an odd-shaped cervix or uterus (which cannot readily house the developing child). Sons of the women who took DES may be at risk as well; research has shown that these men may suffer from a cyst in the testes that impedes sperm production.

As new treatments develop for a range of human ills, they are often put into use with little thought about their effect on fertility. For example, many gynecologists have treated cervical infections by cautery (burning) or cryosurgery (freezing) in the affected area. However, when the women treated in this manner decide they want to have children, some are unsuccessful at conceiving because the doctor has burned or frozen such a large area that the cervix cannot produce its normal mucus.

A variety of drugs for everything from cancer to high blood pressure can lower a man's sperm count. It may seem silly even to discuss the reproductive hazards of such potentially life-saving drugs. Given the choice between suffering and, perhaps, even dying of a serious illness or losing one's fertility, one would almost invariably choose the latter. Many times, however, the choice is made unwittingly or even unnecessarily.

Rather than accepting infertility, a man for whom strong anti-cancer drugs are prescribed can arrange to have some of his healthy predrug sperm frozen. Then, even if he is made sterile by the treatment, he can still "father" a child, since his wife can be inseminated with the preserved sperm. In fact, Kim Casali, the woman who draws the "Love Is" cartoon, gave birth to such a child, conceived from sperm that her husband arranged to freeze before undergoing cancer treatment.

The same freezing techniques could be used by men who worked at jobs that might hamper fertility. But many men are not told about this option until it is too late, until their sperm production system has been hopelessly damaged.

In other instances, there might be alternative ways to treat the illness, only some of which impede fertility. Among the drugs known to affect sperm count are Imuran, prednisone, and certain urinary tract antibacterial medications such as Macrodantin and Furadantin. Sometimes a "cure" for infertility can come about just by switching a man from a sperm-threatening drug to an equally effective medication with no infertility side effects.

In 1982, 1.42 billion prescriptions were written—a 70 percent increase since the U.S. Food and Drug Administration (FDA) started keeping records in 1964. From the standpoint of fertility, it is frightening how little we know about the effects of drugs on our ability to bear children. Consider the drug Tagamet. Introduced in 1977 to treat ulcers, Tagamet has become the best-selling drug in the country, surpassing even the much prescribed Valium. A *New England Journal of Medicine* article revealed that Tagamet depresses a man's sperm count by as much as 43 percent. The problem disappears when the man stops taking Tagamet (actually around three months after, when the entire sperm production and release cycle has had a chance to operate without the drugs). But such findings leave open the worrisome question, How many couples who believe they are hopelessly infertile are only suffering the side effects of a drug? How many who adopt, undergo artificial insemination, or divorce because of the trauma of infertility could have been helped if their problem had been traced to a particular medicine?

Our knowledge gap about the fertility effects of drugs was dramatically illustrated by the recent announcement that the drug Azulfidine may be marketed soon as a male contraceptive. Azulfidine is not a new drug. Since the 1950s men have been taking it for stomach and çolon problems without realizing it hampered fertility!

"The effects of most drugs on fertility have not yet been studied," notes Dr. Sherman Silber, a St. Louis infertility specialist and author of *How to Get Pregnant,* "and they should always be considered culprits, since anything that affects the body's normal functions can affect infertility."

CONTRACEPTIVES

Some drugs and treatments can have devastating effects on fertility even after a person stops using them. Prime among these are contraceptives. In some instances, the techniques that women have chosen to temporarily postpone childbearing have turned against them and caused permanent problems.

The first intrauterine (IUD) for women who had never before been pregnant was introduced in 1970. Currently, 6 percent of the women of reproductive age use IUDs. The small device is inserted into the uterus and remains there until the woman decides to have it removed (for example, in order to become pregnant). It seems to work by producing a mild inflammation of the uterine lining.

The use of an IUD presents a number of potential hazards, however. Since it prevents implantation of the egg in the uterus, but has no effect on implantation in the tubes, the woman might have an ectopic pregnancy, the medical term for an embryo that implants someplace other than in the womb. The most common type of ectopic pregnancy settles in a fallopian tube. If it is not detected early, it can become life-threatening to the woman and has the potential to burst the tube, forever impairing fertility on that side. A woman who later damages her other tube will be completely sterile. This is what caused the infertility of Judy Carr, who went on to become America's first test-tube baby mother.

The IUD sometimes also causes such a severe, permanent irritation to the uterine lining that, even after the device is removed, no egg will be able to implant. In addition, the IUD has been linked to pelvic inflammatory disease (PID), which causes adhesions on the ovaries or blocks the fallopian tubes. In 1974, one type of IUD, the Dalkon shield, was withdrawn from the market because of its tendency to cause PID and septic (infected) spontaneous abortions. A recent study by the National Institutes of Health and the Centers for Disease Control, a federal agency in Atlanta, found that women who used IUDs are 70 percent more likely to develop severe pelvic inflammatory disease than women who use other contraceptive methods.

"Because of the IUD's connection with infections," comments Dr. Martin Quigley, director of the Division of Reproductive Endocrinology and Infertility at the University of Texas Health Science Center in Houston, "I think the IUD is an inappropriate choice of contraception for someone who will want to get pregnant in the future." At the very least, specialists advise that those women with previous pelvic infections not use the IUD.

ABORTION

Abortion, performed on over a million women each year, also affects future fertility in a small number of these women. The number of abortions has naturally increased since our mothers' day, since it was not until 1973 that abortions were legalized. Legalization cut down drastically on the number of abortions being done under unsanitary conditions—the so-called back alley abortions that often resulted in perforation of the uterus, infection, or other hazards to the woman's fertility. Even in the more sanitary conditions of today, a small percentage of women will contract infections from an abortion.

This can happen any time the uterus is exposed to instruments or an atmosphere that could contain bacteria. Such exposure can occur during childbirth itself. Some new mothers experience a postpartum infection; left untreated, it could result in secondary infertility.

Because a smoldering infection can cause scarring of the uterus or tubes, it is important to treat it as soon as possible. A woman who undergoes an abortion or gives birth should contact her doctor immediately if she notices heavy bleeding, runs a high fever, or has an unusual discharge from the vagina after the procedure.

STERILIZATION

While most of the new cases of infertility were unanticipated, one is deliberate. In addition to the growing number of couples who want to have children but cannot conceive, there has been a rapid rise in the number of people who have opted for sterilization. Ten million men have had vasectomies; half a million men are currently being sterilized every year. In recent years, tubal ligation was introduced for women—a simple and more readily reversible form of sterilization than cautery, sealing the tubes with heat. Now 650,000 women per year undergo tubal ligations. About 1 percent of the men and women—or about ten thousand couples a year—change their minds and search for a way to reverse the operations. People request reversal in a variety of situations: when they remarry, when their financial situation improves, or when one of their children dies. Dr. Sherman Silber gives a particularly graphic example of a situation in which a man wanted his vasectomy reversed. Silber's patient, a diplomat with a wife and two children, worked abroad and only returned to the United States two weeks each year. On one of his trips, the diplomat underwent a vasectomy. The next day, his wife was killed in an automobile accident and one child was in critical condition. "He knew just one day after his vasectomy that it had been a terrible mistake," observes Silber.

In another case, a thirty-five-year-old husband and his thirty-two-year-old wife sought Silber's aid. They wanted to have children together, but both had been sterilized in their previous marriages, never dreaming that those marriages were going to fall apart.

Victor Gomel, an infertility specialist at the University of British Columbia in Canada, studied one hundred women who came to him requesting a reversal of their sterilization. Of these, sixty-three of the women made the request because of a change in marital status. Sixteen other women had undergone the sterilization in the postpartum period while still in the hospital after a child's birth; then, tragically, the young child died and the woman wanted the sterilization reversed.

As a result of this study, Gomel advises women to give careful thought to the decision to be sterilized, especially if they are young. (He found that 52 percent of the patients requesting reversal had been under age twenty-five when they were sterilized, 89 percent under thirty). Gomel cautions against undergoing sterilization during the postpartum period, recommending that women use other means of birth control for eight to twelve months before deciding on sterilization.

In Gomel's study, 90 percent of the women said they had not been told about the type of sterilization to be performed or were given no choice. You have a right to this information and should discuss alternative types of sterilization with your doctor. If you are under age thirty-five, you might want to opt for a tubal ligation, in which a small segment of each fallopian tube is excised, rather than for tubal cautery, since the former method is easier to reverse. Or you might want to inquire about the possibility of obtaining a bilateral tubal occlusion, in which silicone rubber plugs are inserted into the fallopian tubes. This procedure, now in the experimental stages, purportedly allows for reversal by removal of the plugs. As Gomel's study hints, it is difficult to predict what twists and turns your life will take and whether a decision for permanent childlessness will continue to fit your life plans.

For men, the *type* of sterilization offered is fairly standard: a vasectomy, a five-minute surgical procedure severing a tube through which the sperm travel from the testicles to the penis. The factor that most affects a reversal attempt is the amount of time that has elapsed since the vasectomy was performed. After a vasectomy, sperm is still produced. It just builds up in the part of the tube nearest the testicles. The pressure created can cause damage to the tubes, preventing the man from recovering normal fertility after vasectomy reversal. Sperm can also escape from the tubes and enter the man's system, causing him to produce antibodies to the sperm. For the diplomat who learned one day later that his vasectomy had been a mistake, the chance for success would be quite high (90 percent). But if a man requests a reversal ten years or more after the original operation, the success rate, even in the hands of a top microsurgeon, drops to 50 percent. The pregnancy rate for reversal of female sterilization can reach as high as 80 percent with micro-surgery.

INFECTIONS

There is no doubt that more women are having sex at a younger age. According to national surveys of metropolitan teenagers, in 1971, 46 percent of the never-married women had sexual inter-course by the time they were 19; by 1979, the figure was 69 per-cent. Along with sexual activity, though, comes the risk of contracting a sexually transmitted pelvic infection, which could lead to infertility by scarring the woman's fallopian tubes or a man's sperm-carrying ducts.

According to researchers at the Centers for Disease Control, one million people suffer from sexually transmitted diseases each year, resulting in infertility in 150,000 to 200,000 of those cases. The leading sexually transmitted infection, lymphogranuloma ve-nereum, caused by the Chlamydia organism, is easily treated, as are gonorrhea and syphillis, but many people do not recognize the symptoms, or ignore them. "The young people of today are only going to feel the problem ten to fifteen years from now when they try to have a child," warns Dr. Paul Weisner, director of V.D. Control Division at the Centers for Disease Control.

New York infertility specialist Dr. Sherwin A. Kaufman, author of *You Can Have a Baby,* has become so concerned about the epidemic of gonorrhea that he advises sexually active women to undergo pelvic examination and gonorrhea culture every few months. Gonorrhea has no overt symptoms in 80 percent of the women it strikes, yet it works silently to scar the fallopian tubes.

LIFESTYLE

Women have made tremendous strides socially, economically, and professionally in the past generation. With new horizons open-ing up to them in education and on the job, many women explore options in other areas of life and postpone having children. The availability of contraceptives gives couples more control over when they will have their first child and how much time they will wait between children.

Since 1965, the proportion of ever-married women under thirty who have never had a child doubled, from 12 percent to 25 percent. In a June 1981 national survey, 20 percent of the over-thirty women having children were giving birth for the first time.

The social trend of postponing childbearing, however, goes against the biological trend in our bodies. For both men and women, peak fertility occurs between the ages of twenty and twenty-five. After age twenty-five, the ability to conceive a child tapers off in both men and women, with the woman's ability decreasing more abruptly. According to the American Fertility Foundation, a twenty-five-year-old woman has a 75 percent chance of conceiving a child after six months of trying. In the late twenties, that drops to 47 percent; in the early thirties, 38 percent; in the late thirties, 25 percent and after age forty, 22 percent.

Although no one likes to face the fact that he or she might have a fertility problem, it is important for a woman in her thirties to seek medical attention fairly rapidly. "A woman who is over age thirty-five and cannot conceive within six months should be evaluated," says Quigley. "Once in her thirties, a woman is subject not only to the undefinable reduction in fertility that occurs with age but also to acquired fertility factors such as greater risk of tubal infection."

As Quigley points out, the decrease in fertility as you age can be traced to a variety of factors: you have had a longer exposure to pollution and a greater chance to encounter fertility hazards in the workplace or as treatment for some illness. You have probably used contraceptives, maybe even an IUD, which is particularly risky for women who later want to become pregnant. You are more likely to suffer from endometriosis, in which small pieces of the endometrium (the uterine lining) flow backward up into the tubes and implant themselves in parts of the abdomen in which they do not belong, hampering conception. What is more, when an older woman finds she has a fertility problem, even a solvable one, there is less time for the cause of and cure for that problem to be discovered.

• *THE THREATS TO FERTILITY TAKE THEIR TOLL*

With the increasing assaults to fertility triggered by our modern environment and lifestyle, one in six couples are finding that they are not able to conceive a child after a year of trying. When you make a decision, as did the Robertsons, that it is time to investigate the cause of your childlessness, it is best to turn to an infertility specialist early on. The medical aspects of diagnosing and treating infertility are becoming increasingly complex as subtle causes of infertility are discovered and new medical techniques are being introduced. The average gynecologist, obstetrician, or urologist, who concentrates on a wide variety of problems in his or her practice, may not have sufficient expertise to investigate your problem in the competent, exhaustive manner it merits.

"Working with an infertility problem is like doing detective work," notes Dr. H. M. Hasson, an associate professor at the Rush Medical College in Chicago. "The couple might be lucky and you'll hit upon the problem right away—the medical equivalent of learning that the butler did it. But it also could be something that you don't find until the later stages of the investigation. You must do it methodically. The worst thing a doctor can do is just give you fertility drugs without looking into the causes."

An infertility specialist will generally initially see the husband and wife together, asking them both many questions about their medical, marital, and sexual history. Although some of the questions will be horribly intrusive ("How often do you make love?" "In what position?" "Have you ever achieved a pregnancy with someone other than your spouse?"), they are not inappropriate. Facts such as the wife having undergone an abortion in the past or the husband having impregnated a former lover can provide a crucial clue to the doctor. If you will not feel comfortable discussing these matters with the doctor in the presence of your spouse, then think about going over them with your spouse before visiting the doctor. At the very least, if you choose to avoid sharing the information with your spouse, phone the doctor and explain the facts, asking him or her, if you like, to keep them confidential. Sharing sensitive information with your doctor can save you time, money, and, occasionally, physical pain, by avoiding the use of unnecessary tests.

The doctor will talk to you about your lovemaking technique because couples sometimes unwittingly hamper fertility by their sexual style. K-Y jelly and Surgilube, for example, kill sperm. If a woman gets up immediately after making love, many sperm will leak out. If she douches, that can destroy the sperm. It is best for the woman to lie still for half an hour after intercourse to increase the chances of the sperm reaching the egg.

Some couples think that "saving up" sperm will give them a better chance at getting pregnant. But abstaining from intercourse for more than four days before the woman's fertile time can adversely affect the mobility of sperm. On the other hand, having sex too frequently can temporarily further lower a man's low sperm count.

In addition to the questions the doctor will ask you and the advice he or she will give you about the technique of intercourse, the doctor will do a physical exam of both of you (or, if he or she deals primarily with women's problems, the husband will be sent to a urologist for a physical). This exam, often accompanied by urine and blood tests, will tell whether there is some infection or other general disease process at work in your body that could be interfering with your fertility. The doctor will also check for any current infections in the reproductive system. For example, nonspecific urethritis can cause temporary infertility apparently by lowering the man's sperm count and altering the shape of the sperm. A high dosage of antibiotics can eliminate the troublesome infection. If the results of these tests are normal, the doctor will then begin a special workup on you and your spouse.

The American Fertility Society has prepared a booklet for doctors, "How to Organize a Basic Study of the Infertile Couple." You might want to read it for a better understanding of the tests the doctor will be proposing and why he or she is suggesting them. The booklet is available for one dollar from the American Fertility

Society, 1608 13th Avenue South, Suite 101, Birmingham, Alabama 35246.

Throughout testing and treatment, it is important to ask questions of your doctor to understand more fully what is going on. Many couples have unbased fears about the procedures that can be cleared up by obtaining more information.

It is not always easy to pin down a busy infertility specialist. But you have a legal right to know what will be done to you, why, how, and what alternatives exist. Massachusetts infertility counselor Ellen Bresnick finds that the better the understanding patients have of the rationale for tests and therapies, the more capable they are of coping emotionally.

With some doctors, the infertility workup can last up to a year or two because certain tests must be performed at specific times during the woman's menstrual cycle. Other doctors coordinate the tests, performing a number each month so that the investigation takes three to six months. Let your doctor know your feelings about how you would like to proceed and what sort of timetable is most comfortable for you.

"Some couples really want to quit and initiate adoption but don't know how," relates Barbara Eck Menning, founder of Resolve, a national self-help group for infertile couples. "If they are ready to quit and the doctor pursues the investigation, stress can crack the relationship. And then they may have nothing, not even each other."

Many couples feel the worst part of infertility is the waiting period while endless investigations occur, with them not knowing whether or not they can be helped. Luckily, advances have been made that allow doctors more readily to give definitive diagnoses. In 1958, there was no known explanation for the problem in 24 percent of all infertile couples. Now, a specific diagnosis can be made in all but 8 percent of infertile couples.

3 ❧ Investigating and Enhancing Your Fertility

If you and your spouse are among the unlucky 15 percent of the population who cannot get pregnant after a year of trying, there are a wide range of diagnostic tests, ranging from simple to complex, that you can undertake. You should systematically undergo any that might reveal the cause of your problem until you have exhausted all possibilities or decided that you do not wish to proceed further. On the basis of the test results, your physician may be able to enhance your fertility through the use of drugs, surgery, or other treatments.

As you and your spouse search for the cause of your infertility, you should both undergo investigations at the same time. For many years, it was assumed that if a couple could not have a baby, it was the woman's fault. Even though it is now known that the male contributes to the problem in 40 percent to 60 percent of all infertile couples, some doctors focus their evaluation on the woman first.

"Nothing bothers me more than a wife having gone through a complete evaluation, including biopsies, laparoscopies, hysterosalpingograms, perhaps even several trials of clomiphene, only subsequently to find out that her husband has a severely low sperm count," says Dr. Martin Quigley, Director of the Division of Reproductive Endocrinology and Infertility at the University of Texas Health Science Center in Houston. "A semen analysis is cheap, easy, painless, and has no complications. I think the semen analysis needs to be done either first, or at the latest, simultaneous with the initiation of the wife's evaluation."

Once the status of the man's sperm count is learned, the evaluation of his wife can proceed. "If the sperm count is the slightest bit low some doctors tell the couple they just can't have any children together," charges St. Louis infertility specialist Dr. Sherman Silber. "The doctors overlook the fact that 10 percent of men of proven fertility have sperm counts in the low range. Even though men with very low counts—say, around ten million—have less of a statistical chance of getting their wives pregnant, they still can do it with time, patience, and appropriate treatment of their wives to boost the chance of a pregnancy."

According to Silber, evaluation and treatment of one spouse alone is "a misperception that can result in no conception." Infertility is rarely absolute or limited to one partner. Since a *combination* of complex processes within both the husband and wife prompts conception, sometimes a fertility shortcoming on the part of one spouse can be overcome by a high degree of fertility in the other. For example, a man with a low sperm count might have no trouble fathering a child if he is married to a woman with perfectly regular ovulation and more-conducive-than average cervical mucus. Likewise, a woman with only one fallopian tube functioning might have a better chance of getting pregnant if she is married to a man with a high quality of sperm. This is why some people who have had no trouble conceiving a child in a previous marriage sometimes have difficulty when they remarry. In fact, Napoleon and Josephine were a classic case of borderline fertility. Although unable to have children together, they were both fertile with other mates.

"Most infertile couples represent a combination of problems in the husband and wife," Sibler observes. Overattention to one spouse's problem can cause neglect of an easily treated problem in the other spouse.

"A preliminary evaluation, including a postcoital test, hysterosalpingogram, semen analysis, and some test for ovulation (either a blood test or an endometrial biopsy) can be accomplished within a period of, at most, eight weeks," notes Quigley. "At the end of that time the couple should be told what the preliminary results are, what the remainder of the evaluation would entail, and

---

CHECKLIST OF COMMON INFERTILITY TESTS

A variety of medical tests are available to determine the cause of a person's infertility. Although a particular individual would probably not need to undergo all the available tests, this checklist is presented so that you and your physician can determine which tests you might require. The tests are discussed in detail in this chapter and the following one.

THE WOMAN'S LIST

_____ Physical
_____ Basal body temperature charting
_____ Mid-cycle pelvic exam
_____ Analysis of cervical mucus
_____ Endometrial biopsy or radioimmunoassays
_____ Urine tests and/or blood tests for hormone levels
_____ Postcoital test
_____ Hysterosalpingography
_____ Laparoscopy
_____ Chromosome testing (in rare instances)
_____ Human leukocyte antigen (HLA) testing (in rare instances)

---

what the ultimate chance of success would be. I have found couples who are told that following ovulation induction with Clomid they have a 50 percent chance of pregnancy and don't want to put up with the hassle, and I have had couples who would undergo a major tubal operation for a 5 percent chance of fertility. I think that is a decision the couple must make and they can only do that when they have been given a reasonable idea of what the remainder of the infertility evaluation would entail, what the treat-

---

CHECKLIST OF COMMON INFERTILITY TESTS

THE MAN'S LIST

____ Physical
____ Examination of size of testicles
____ Examination of testicles for varicose vein in spermatic
cord
____ Analysis of quantity of semen
____ Analysis of quantity of sperm
____ Analysis of motility (speed) of sperm
____ Analysis of morphology (shape) or sperm
____ Vasogram X ray
____ Testicular biopsy
____ Urine tests and/or blood tests for hormone levels
____ Hamster egg penetration test
____ Mucus penetration test
____ Blood test for sperm antibodies
____ Chromosome testing (in rare instances)
____ Human leukocyte antigen (HLA) testing (in rare
instances)

---

ment would entail, and what their ultimate chance of becoming pregnant would be."

• *THE WOMAN'S INFERTILITY WORKUP*

An invaluable compass in the search for a cause of female infertility is a simple, inexpensive procedure: charting the Basal Body Temperature (BBT). The complex story of the changes taking place monthly in a woman's body are told graphically by her temperature. In a normal cycle, the woman's temperature is three tenths of a degree to a full degree lower during the first half of the cycle, beginning with the first day of her period, than it is during the second half. This can be a contrast of 97.4 degrees Fahrenheit or lower to 98 degrees or higher. A sudden rise in temperature midway through the cycle indicates that ovulation has taken place, usually around twenty-four hours before the rise. (Consequently, a woman's most fertile time is twenty-four hours before the temperature rise—unfortunately, such a determination can only be made retrospectively.)

A basal body temperature is taken orally first thing in the morning, every morning. Since any activity raises the temperature, you should shake down a thermometer before you go to bed and take your temperature upon awakening before even getting out of bed. A special oral basal body temperature thermometer is available that covers only the degrees from 95 to 100; its lengthy intervals allow you to easily tell the temperature to the nearest one tenth of a degree. You plot your temperature on a graph and make note of any factors (such as a cold, lack of sleep, or medication) that might have thrown your temperature off that day. Some doctors also have the couple put a circle or X on the chart indicating the days they have made love. If you and your husband engage in extensive business travel or otherwise make love infrequently, your infertility problems may be caused by nothing more than failing to make love on the days when you are most fertile.

If you are ovulating, the graph will be divided into two distinct halves, with temperatures at a lower level in the first half of the cycle. If you do not ovulate that month, your temperature will vary in little ups and downs throughout the month with no dramatic distinction between the first and second half. The graph will disclose whether there is a shortened second half of the cycle (known as an inadequate luteal phase), in which the first half of the cycle (with low temperatures) lasts for fourteen days but the second half (with the high temperatures) lasts only five to twelve days. This is evidence that the ovary is not sending out sufficient progesterone, which in turn affects the uterine lining and could cause infertility by preventing a fertilized egg from implanting itself.

A woman's cycle can vary from month to month and can be

thrown off by many things, including the uncertainty and novelty of the infertility workup itself. Do not let your reading of a one-month basal body temperature graph panic you. It usually takes three to four months of charting plus the eye of an experienced infertility expert to read the nuances in the basal body temperature chart.

Other painless tests are also available to determine whether a woman's cycle is on the appropriate course. If ovulation is occurring, a midcycle pelvic exam should show that the woman's cervix is open more widely. The doctor might take a sample of the mucus during a pelvic exam to test its elasticity and microscopic appearance for other clues to whether ovulation is occurring. Within twelve hours of ovulation, the mucus becomes sticky and impenetrable.

Specialists disagree as to what additional tests are necessary to assess a woman's cycle. Some advocate an endometrial biopsy, where a snippet of the uterine lining is scraped off in the second half of the cycle. Others believe this test is unnecessary unless the temperature chart is equivocal or a progesterone deficiency is suspected in the second half of a seemingly normal cycle. The endometrial biopsy is an office procedure that women find to be painful. As an alternative, sophisticated blood tests called radioimmunoassays can be done to assess the progesterone level during the second half of the cycle. This technique may be more costly than the biopsy, but you might want to ask about it if your physician is suggesting an endometrial biospy.

If these tests show that the woman is ovulating, the physician will order other blood or urine tests to monitor the levels of certain hormones—such as prolactin or testosterone. This additional testing will help him or her determine which important link in the cycle has broken down and will help determine what medicines might repair or replace that link.

Other simple tests of ovulation are also on the horizon. At the Monell Chemical Sense Center in Philadelphia, chemists James Kostelc and George Preti have been analyzing the changes in a woman's saliva that occur during each month. They found that levels of a substance called N-dodecanol exceeded normal levels by ten times at ovulation. "Perhaps in the future, this may lead to a self-administered fertility test," says Preti. Such a test would consist of a special paper that would change color in contact with a woman's saliva if she were ovulating.

A test that provides both information about a woman's cycle and her husband's sperm is the postcoital test, performed around the time of ovulation, the thirteenth or fourteenth day of the cycle. The name of this test has confused many people. "We were prepared for anything," recalls Marsha Sheinfeld, president of the Chicago chapter of Resolve, "including making love on the doctor's examining table." The test does take place after lovemaking, but the intercourse takes place at home, with the woman presenting herself to the doctor from two to twelve hours later (specialists vary in their opinion as to the best time to perform the test). The doctor then performs a pelvic exam, taking secretions from different levels in the cervical canal (and sometimes within the uterus as well). These secretions are analyzed under a microscope to determine whether a sufficient number of sperm are making their way through the woman's genital tract. (The cervical mucus test described earlier can also be performed at this time.)

If the woman's cycle is normal, yet few or no sperm show up in the mucus, there may be a problem with the quantity or quality of the husband's sperm. (An analysis of the husband's semen will shed further light on the issue.) In rare instances, though, it might indicate an immunologic reaction (where the woman has formed antibodies to her partner's sperm) or an infection—both of which can be investigated by further, painless tests. The immunologic reaction is gauged by mixing a drop of the woman's blood with some of her husband's sperm to determine the reaction and by testing for antisperm antibodies or agglutinatins antibodies in the cervical mucus itself. Infections such as those caused by T mycoplasmas (thought by some specialists to play an obscure role in many cases of infertility and chronic habitual abortion) can be diagnosed by a culture of the wife's cervical secretions or the husband's semen.

If, though, the woman is ovulating regularly and the postcoital tests reveal sufficient quantities of high-quality sperm gaining entry through the cervix, the physician may suspect that a blockage in the fallopian tubes is impeding the progress of the sperm toward the egg or that endometriosis is hampering the woman's fertility.

The fallopian tubes serve several functions. The delicate fimbria (the ends of the tubes closest to the ovaries) reach over to cover up the ovarian follicle prior to the release of the egg. The hairlike cilia inside the tubes and the muscular contractions transport the egg down the tube. The secretions inside the tube can nourish a fertilized egg on its several-day journey down a tube en route to implantation in the uterus.

The most common cause of tubal problems is infection, which can cause scarring inside the tube or adhesions at the entryway to the tube. As described earlier, some women whose mothers took DES have tubal problems, as do some women who suffer from endometriosis.

When a woman has endometriosis, pieces of the endometrium, the lining of the uterus, flow backward up into the tubes and implant themselves in parts of the abdomen in which they do not belong. Most commonly, they implant on the ovaries. Women with endometriosis are only half as likely to get pregnant as women in the general population.

Analysis of tubal functioning is still relatively crude. The tests that have been devised so far focus on whether the tube is open or closed. One diagnostic tool, the Rubin test, has been in use since 1919. It is an office procedure, performed during the first half of the cycle. The doctor inserts a thin tube into the cervix and pumps some carbon dioxide into the uterus. If at least one of the tubes is open, the gas will pass through the tube. There are two signs that passage has occurred. First, there will be a drop in the pressure gauge connected to the gas. Second, when the woman sits up, she will feel pain in one or both shoulders, as the gas continues its journey. Both of these things indicate that at least one tube is open and, thus, an alternative explanation for the infertility must be sought.

However, just because neither of these two signs of gas passage occurs does not necessarily mean that the tubes are closed. The tube may appear closed because of a temporary spasm—for example, if the woman is not fully relaxed when undergoing the test. In about 32 percent of the cases, tubes that seem closed on the Rubin test are found to be open on a subsequent X ray. For that reason, most doctors skip the Rubin test entirely and proceed directly with hysterosalpingography, an X ray of the uterus and tubes that involves introducing a dye (rather than carbon dioxide gas) into the uterus. The X ray provides more precise information than the Rubin test since it can show uterine lesions and detect whether one or both tubes are blocked. However, even the X ray may not give a completely accurate picture. As with the Rubin test, a temporary tubal spasm may erroneously give the impression that a tube is permanently blocked. For that reason, Dr. Melvin L. Taymor, clinical professor of obstetrics and gynecology at the Harvard Medical School, advises doctors never to contemplate tubal surgery on the basis of a single X ray.

The most intrusive test in the woman's workup is the laparoscopy, a surgical procedure that allows the doctor to directly view the organs in the abdominal and pelvic area. For the test, performed under anesthesia in a hospital, the doctor makes a one-half-inch incision in or just below the woman's navel and inserts a laparoscope, a telescopelike instrument through which he or she can make an examination. According to the American Fertility Society, of the women with infertility due to unknown causes, laparoscopy will reveal a definitive diagnosis 30 percent of the time.

Through the laparoscope, the doctor looks for adhesions that could be blocking the tubes or interfering with the ability of the sperm to move toward the ovaries. The doctor may inject a dye into the uterus and watch whether it can travel through the tubes.

The doctor will also examine the ovaries for bubblelike appearance (indicating that ovulation is not occurring) or adhesions (which could interfere with ovulation). Laparoscopy is also the only way to make a definitive diagnosis of endometriosis. The doctor does so by searching for evidence of endometrial tissue in areas on the tubes or ovaries or elsewhere in the pelvic area (other than in its normal home, the uterus).

In addition to its telescopic powers, the laparoscope has a tiny scissorslike instrument at its end. If the woman's internal problems are minor (such as mild adhesions), the doctor can correct the problem during the diagnostic laparoscopy. If the problems are more extensive, the woman will be scheduled for a subsequent operation.

For some couples, the infertility problem is not an inability to conceive. Although the woman can achieve a pregnancy, the fetus does not develop to term, but rather spontaneously aborts. The reason for the miscarriage must be pinpointed so that steps can be taken to protect future pregnancies.

About 15 percent of all pregnancies end in miscarriage. Half of the first trimester miscarriages are due to chromosomal abnormalities, discussed in greater detail in Chapter Four. Between 10 percent and 15 percent of the early miscarriages are caused by an abnormality of the uterus, such as an odd shape or the presence of benign tumors within the uterus.

An incompetent cervix can lead to miscarriages later in the pregnancy, during the fourth to sixth month. In such instances, the cervix is not strong enough to hold the fetus in place as it develops through the pregnancy.

A variety of diagnostic techniques are available to pinpoint the cause of a woman's fertility. Some of these techniques themselves can help lead to a pregnancy. The passage of dye through the tubes in a hysterosalpingogram can clear them of minor blockages, enhancing the possibility of conception. For other women, though, the diagnostic tests merely prepare the blueprint upon which treatment is then based. In general, when a final diagnosis is made of a large number of infertile women, 40 percent are found to have tubal problems, 30 percent have ovulatory problems, 15 percent have endometriosis, and 5 percent have cervical problems.

• *TREATMENT OF THE WOMAN*

At various points in the infertility workup, the doctor may stop and try a particular treatment. Depending on the specific infertility problem, the doctor will recommend drugs, surgery, or a combination of both.

A tremendous amount of progress has been made in recent years in the treatment of women who have ovulatory problems.

Infertile couples are probably most familiar with clomiphene citrate, sold under the trade names of Clomid and Serophene, which stimulates the release of the hormones FSH and LH, causing a follicle to grow and an egg to be expelled. Clomiphene citrate is generally prescribed for women whose bodies produce some of these hormones, but just not enough. It improves the quality and regulation of ovulation and is also helpful for a luteal phase defect.

Ironically, the scientists who developed clomiphene citrate were trying to produce a contraceptive. Although the drug has contraceptive effects in animals, in humans it enhances fertility. After taking clomiphene citrate, 70 percent of women appear to ovulate. According to the records of 5157 women taking the drug, 35 percent became pregnant. About 10 percent of the women taking Clomid have a multiple pregnancy (generally twins).

Much stronger substances, gonadotropins, are used when clomiphene citrate fails or when the woman is not a good candidate for clomiphene citrate because her body does not produce FSH and LH.

Human menopausal gonadotropin (HMG), refined from the urine of women who have gone through menopause, is rich in FSH and LH. When production of Pergonal (the trade name for HMG) began in Italy around twenty years ago, a prime source for the urine was the Catholic convents. The older nuns, precluded by their religious vows from having their own children, were delighted to play a role in another woman's pregnancy.

HMG stimulates the ovaries so that a follicle matures. Another substance, human chorionic gonadotrophin (HCG), similar to LH, is administered midcycle to actually trigger the ovulation. HCG is also purified from the urine of women but, in this case, it is the urine of pregnant women.

Extremely careful monitoring is necessary when a woman uses gonadotropins. These substances are so powerful that they can overstimulate the ovary, causing it to enlarge, painfully swelling up the abdominal cavity and sometimes causing blood pressure to fall. In severe cases, the woman will need to be hospitalized.

To avoid this harrowing side effect, the doctor should order blood tests to monitor the estrogen level in your blood (a clue to the stage of ripening of the follicle). If there is too much estrogen, the doctor should skip the administration of HCG in that cycle rather than run the risk of overstimulating the ovary. Recent advances in the use of ultrasound (a process whereby sound waves are bounced off the pelvic area, then picked up on a computer screen) allow skilled ultrasound technicians, to make judgments about the size of the developing follicle and decide about HCG use. Even with extremely careful monitoring, however, overstimulation occurs in 1 to 3 percent of the women who use Pergonal.

It is important to undergo Pergonal therapy only with a doctor who is thoroughly familiar with the drug. Even the manufacturer has issued the warning that in light of its potential side effects, "unless a physician is willing to devote considerable time to these patients and be familiar with and conduct the necessary laboratory studies, he should not use Pergonal®. . . ."

If gonadotropin therapy is used properly, about 30 percent of the patients begin to ovulate and 50 to 70 percent of those ovulating become pregnant. The risk of multiple pregnancies with HMG has been reported as high—around 20 percent. About 4 percent of births are triplets or more.

An alternative to Pergonal and HCG may be a hormone called gonadotropin release hormone (GnRH), which acts directly on the pituitary gland, making it produce the other hormones necessary for fertility. The difficulty with GnRH, which is being used experimentally, is that it must be injected into the bloodstream in short bursts, once every one and a half hours for two weeks. Dr. Samuel S. C. Yen and his colleagues at the University of California at San Diego have developed a special GnRH -administering intravenous pump that women may wear while they go about their normal activities.

Other promising research tentatively suggests that the drug bromocriptine (usual trade name: Parlodel) might sometimes be helpful for ovulatory problems. Women who are pregnant or nursing have a high level of the hormone prolactin in their bodies, which decreases the level of FSH and LH, the hormones necessary for ovulation. Some infertile women, however, also have this high prolactin level, and the drug bromocriptine is extremely useful in lowering the prolactin level. This drug does not appear to be helpful to women who have a normal level of prolactin but do not ovulate.

Bromocriptine is also used by some doctors for treatment of luteal phase deficiency, a syndrome in which the second part of the menstrual cycle is shortened and the uterine lining does not develop sufficiently to sustain an embryo. Medical attention has focused on this problem only recently and the best method of treatment has not yet been determined. Doctors may offer progesterone, clomiphene citrate, or Pergonal.

If you are taking bromocriptine, notify your doctor if your period is late. The drug should not be used during pregnancy since it appears to affect the fetus, leading to a greater number of abnormalities and stillbirths than is in the population at large.

A woman whose cervical mucus is hostile to her husband's sperm is sometimes helped by a small dose of the hormone estrogen on days ten to fourteen of her cycle. Since the problem may be that the mucus is too acidic, the doctor may alternatively recommend that the woman use an alkaline douche. Some doctors are finding that guaifenesin, an expectorant that is an ingredient in some cough medicines (for example, Robitussin), seems to help abnormal cervical mucus.

In the rare instances when a woman's immunological reaction to her husband's sperm seems to be affecting fertility, the couple is advised to avoid introducing the husband's sperm into the wife's body for a period of time, generally from sixty days to six months. The couple should not have oral sex and should have genital sex only when using a condom. At the end of the allotted time span, another immunological test is performed. Ideally, the woman's body will have stopped producing the destructive antibodies at that time. If not, condom therapy will continue for an additional period of time.

For some women, infertility is a result of the Stein-Leventhal syndrome (the polycystic ovary syndrome), which is usually diagnosed by the absence of menstruation, enlarged ovaries, excessive hair growth (for example on the lip or stomach), and, in some cases, obesity. For reasons researchers do not entirely understand, surgical removal of a tiny triangular-shaped piece of the ovary sometimes helps these women conceive. But the surgery itself may cause an additional infertility problem: pelvic adhesions. At the very least, drugs to induce ovulation should be tried before surgery is even suggested.

Dr. Melvin Taymor of Harvard is currently involved in the clinical trials of a new drug, a pure FSH, for women who have polycystic ovaries. If his research establishes the efficacy of the drug, the approval of the Food and Drug Administration will be sought to allow the marketing of the medication.

For the woman with endometriosis, various types of drugs and surgery are also available. In endometriosis, pieces of the uterine lining that have deposited themselves outside the uterus respond to the woman's hormones and grow.

One way to treat the condition is to fool the body into thinking it is pregnant (at which time the monthly cycle of growing and bleeding stops). Physicians prescribe continuous use of birth control pills to attain this pseudopregnancy.

A newer treatment for endometriosis, danazol (usual trade name: Danocrine), operates on a different principle. It blocks the production of FSH and LH, stopping ovulation and fooling the body into thinking it has entered menopause. Without these hormones, the endometrial tissue will not grow. Creating a pseudomenopause instead of a pseudopregnancy is favored by doctors as more effective. The side effects of danazol, though, include menopausallike symptoms (hot flashes, acne, hair loss), which are reversed once the drug is discontinued.

Surgery is also used in some cases to combat endometriosis. During laparoscopy, the doctor may be able to cauterize some of the growths. Often more radical surgery is necessary, however. There has been a trend in recent years toward following surgery with danazol to make absolutely sure that no misplaced endometrial tissue remains. However, a paper presented at a recent American Fertility Society meeting challenges that approach. It points out that the time a woman who has had endometriosis is most likely to get pregnant is soon after she recovers from surgery.

Putting such a woman on a drug that stops ovulation (by simulating pregnancy or menapause) for months after surgery may deprive the woman of her most likely opportunity to become pregnant.

When the pelvic problem is not endometriosis but adhesions from past infections or past operations, the woman is usually required to undergo surgery. Minor adhesions can sometimes be removed during laparoscopy, but more extensive damage might require tuboplasty, the surgical repair of the tubes. Some doctors offer patients the option of microsurgery, a process whereby the doctor uses an operating microscope to magnify the organs he or she is viewing in the woman's pelvic area. This allows the surgeon to do a more finely tuned job of removing adhesions and repairing the fallopian tubes. The chance of pregnancy after reconstruction of the tubes is about 30 percent.

Various treatments are also available for women who have experienced repeated spontaneous abortions. The removal of benign tumors from the interior of the uterus leads to a 50 percent rate of viable pregnancies. Surgery can be used to correct an abnormally shaped uterus. An incompetent cervix can be remedied by stitches that hold the cervix closed until the time of delivery, when they are removed.

New treatments for women are on the horizon. A number of doctors are using laser surgery to remove adhesions and treat endometriosis. In Japan and Australia, physicians are experimenting with artificial fallopian tubes made of polyurethane. These presumably could be used by a woman whose own tubes have been hopelessly blocked by disease or have been removed during ectopic pregnancies.

Researchers in infertility at the National Institutes of Health have conducted experiments on monkeys with blocked fallopian tubes. The scientists remove the egg from the monkey's ovary and transfer it to the lower part of the tube, where it can come in contact with the fertilizing sperm. There is a 16 percent pregnancy rate in monkeys after such an egg transfer.

Already, one infertility specialist claims to have achieved a pregnancy in a female patient in a similar manner. The woman had undergone a tubal ligation after having three children. When she remarried, she decided to have the sterilization reversed, but her physician advised her against it. The specialist agreed to try to reconstruct her tubes, but at the same time offered her the option of transferring an egg from her ovary to the lower part of her fallopian tube that was connected to her uterus. She was given Clomid on days five through nine of her cycle. At 10:00 P.M. of the twelfth day of her cycle, she was artificially inseminated with sperm from her husband and then at 8:00 A.M. the next morning she underwent surgery. During the operation, the surgeon removed an egg and transferred it to the lower part of the fallopian tube. He also reversed her sterilization. Nine months later she gave birth to a healthy seven-pound four-ounce boy.

• *THE MAN'S INFERTILITY WORKUP*

Research on the causes and treatment of male infertility has lagged far behind that investigating women. Historically, when a marriage was barren, it was viewed as the woman's fault. In the 1950s, men were thought to be the cause of a couple's infertility in only 10 percent of the cases; now, with more sophisticated testing, it has been learned that the man is the source of the problem in 40 percent of the cases and has a contributing problem in an additional 20 percent.

The prime diagnostic measures in the male infertility workup are the history, physical, and semen analysis.

The man will be asked a variety of questions about childhood diseases (since some, such as mumps during puberty, can cause infertility), operations in the pelvic area (occasionally, doctors performing hernia operations have accidentally severed the vas deferens), or venereal infections (which can scar a man's tubes, thus making it difficult or impossible for the sperm to be ejaculated in the seminal fluid).

During the physical, the doctor will examine the testicles for size and appearance. Testicles smaller than one inch in diameter signal a possible difficulty in sperm production. A varicose vein in the spermatic cord (known as a varicocele) can also cause infertility.

Although many men with varicoceles are fertile, for some men they interfere with sperm production, lowering the sperm count and causing the production of irregularly shaped sperm. In fact, in a 1973 study of 1,294 infertile men by Dr. Richard Amelar and Dr. Lawrence Dubin of the New York University School of Medicine, varicoceles were the leading problem, present in 39 percent of the patients. According to Amelar and Dubin, about 15 percent of all men have varicoceles, with sperm production being affected in two thirds of them.

For the sperm count, the doctor will ask the man to masturbate into a jar and bring the sample to the office for testing within two to three hours. In addition to checking the quantity, motility (speed), and morphology (shape) of the sperm, the technician will determine whether the sperm agglutinate (stick together in groups), making it hard for a single sperm to break away and fertilize an egg.

A relatively new test of sperm is also offered in some clinics. Technicians judge the fertilizing potential of the man's sperm by testing whether the sperm can penetrate a hamster egg that has had its protective outer layers removed. The egg dies out soon after penetration, so there is no chance of its developing into a part human, part hamster (although some scientists jokingly refer to the test as the "humster" test).

Other new tests of the fertilizing power of the sperm involve introducing sperm into a small pool of bovine mucus or a newly developed artificial mucus and watching under a microscope whether the sperm has the power to traverse the mucus.

The infertility specialist may also do some tests on the semen, the liquid in which the sperm travels, to determine whether it has the proper traits to transport the sperm to the female cervix. "Chemicals in the seminal fluid protect the sperm from the acid secretions in the vagina," explains Dr. Amelar. The volume of the semen is also important. If the volume of semen is low, the semen does not sufficiently protect the sperm and carry it to its destination. Too high a volume of semen can also be problematic, since it may dilute the sperm.

A doctor should not make any definitive pronouncements about a man's fertility on the basis of a single sperm and semen analysis. Because a man normally makes new sperm every day and the quantity varies, the doctor should request three or more samples, taken at least two weeks apart.

If a few or no sperm are found in analyzing these samples, the doctor may suggest a testicular biopsy. In this procedure, a one-quarter-inch incision is made in the scrotum and a tissue sample is taken from the testicles. Although it is relatively simple to remove the tissue, the interpretation of its appearance under the microscope is quite difficult and should be undertaken only by an expert. The microscopic analysis should reveal sperm in several stages of production from early precursor cells to full development, thus identifying a problem in a particular stage of the production. If, notwithstanding adequate production of sperm, few or no sperm are being ejaculated, the doctor can reason that there is some blockage preventing the sperm from making their escape. Although most doctors think the absence of problems with production of sperm is sufficient evidence of blockage, some confirm it with an X ray (called a vasogram) that involves passing a dye through the sperm duct.

In relatively few instances of male infertility, the cause may be hormonal. To determine whether such a problem exists, the doctor may order some special blood tests to determine whether there are abnormalities in the pituitary, hypothalamus, adrenal glands, thyroid, or testes. Another rare problem the doctor may test for is a husband's immune reaction (or allergy) to his own sperm (odd as that may seem). Although sperm usually reside within the man in tubules in the testes, in some men the sperm escape and enter the bloodstream. The man's body, thinking the sperm are foreign invaders (like an infection), begins to destroy the sperm.

In general, when a final diagnosis is made on a large number of infertile men, 39 percent have varicoceles, 14 percent have testicular failure, 12 percent have semen volume problems, 9 percent have endocrine problems, and 8 percent have ductal obstructions. Rarer problems include sperm agglutination in eight infertile men in one thousand and high sperm density in two of one thousand infertile men.

• *TREATMENT OF THE MAN*

While a woman is born with all the eggs she will ever need, a man is constantly producing sperm. So when a man's sperm count is low, or there are irrregularities in the sperm themselves, the doctor tries to determine which aspects of the patient's general health and environment may be taking their toll on sperm production.

Sperm are produced optimally when the temperature of the testicles is less than 95 degrees Fahrenheit. If a man has a sperm count in the low range of normal, excessive heat may be enough to push him into the infertile range. In such a case, the doctor will advise him to take showers rather than hot baths, wear boxer rather than jockey shorts, and to try to avoid sitting in one spot all day (such as at a desk or behind the wheel of a truck). The doctor will also advise the man to switch to other drugs if he is taking Imuran, prednisone, Furadantin or other drugs that commonly interfere with the production of sperm.

If, once all the environmental sperm suppressors (such as drugs and heat) are removed, the man still produces few sperm, there is very little that can be done for him. For one thing, it is more difficult to get a man's body to produce sperm than it is to get a woman's body to ovulate an already produced egg. In addition, there has not been the same degree of attention paid to research about hormonal treatments for men as there has been for women. This will undoubtedly be an area of stepped-up effort now that the problems of male infertility are finally beginning to be systematically addressed.

Doctors are, however, experimenting with the use of certain hormones on men to stimulate sperm production. Some of these hormones are the same ones that are used to help infertile women. Clomiphene citrate, although not approved by the FDA for use by men, has purportedly helped some men achieve a greater sperm output and appears to offer a pregnancy rate of 20 to 30 percent. Likewise, HMG and HCG are advocated by some doctors for men with sperm counts below ten million per cubic centimeter. Although about 50 percent of the men show improvement, only about 10 percent achieve conception. A more controversial treatment for low sperm counts is the male hormone testosterone. Although testosterone depresses the sperm count even further, the doctors hope to create a rebound effect where the sperm reaches new heights after temporary suppression. Unfortunately, many men are not helped at all by this approach and some end up with no sperm production at all.

The quest to raise men's sperm counts induces some doctors to use a modern-day equivalent of black magic medicine. Doctors will administer thyroid medicine to men (even in instances where the thyroid is not the cause of the problem) or administer an antibiotic treatment when there is no evidence of infection.

Dr. Sherman Silber deplores this approach. He charges that even when some men do manage to achieve conception after such treatments, there is no evidence that the treatment per se is the cause of the improvement. The man might have been part of the percentage that spontaneously achieve conception even without treatment. At a recent meeting of the American Fertility Society, Silber called for more controlled studies before subjecting men to these witchcraftlike remedies.

For other male infertility problems, however, a fairly high, well-documented success rate has been achieved. Take the case of a varicocele—a varicose vein in the spermatic cord. The varicocele is thought to harm sperm by causing warmer blood and toxins to collect in the groin. In a simple procedure a surgeon can tie off this vein through a small incision made just above the scrotum. By three months later, sperm production is generally improved; 40 to 60 percent of the men achieve conception. Other treatments for varicoceles currently being developed include the insertion of a small silicone balloon in the faulty vein or the use of a special scrotal supporter designed to cool the testicles.

When a testicular biopsy signals a blockage interfering with the release of sperm, the surgeon will operate to remove the ductal impediment. Or, if the man is infertile due to the earlier sterilization, the surgeon can operate to reverse the vasectomy. The chances of successful surgery and a subsequent pregnancy increase in the hands of a competent microsurgeon, a doctor who operates while viewing the ducts or vas deferens through a microscope.

A low volume of seminal fluid is sometimes successfully treated by inseminating the wife with her husband's sperm to give the sperm a head start toward their rendezvous with the egg. This is known as AIH, artificial insemination by husband. The husband will be asked to ejaculate into a specimen jar. The wife will bring the specimen to her doctor's office and assume the position for a routine pelvic exam. The physician will inject the semen into the cervical canal and ask the woman to remain lying down for ten to thirty minutes or he or she will put the semen in a cervical cup that the woman will wear, like a diaphragm, for the following four to six hours.

AIH is sometimes used when the man has a low sperm count. Because the greatest concentration of sperm is found in the first portion of the semen, the man will be asked to ejaculate into two specimen jars. The first one, which usually contains the highest concentration of semen, will be used for the artificial insemination. This split ejaculate technique can also be achieved through normal intercourse by having the male withdraw after the first few spurts of ejaculation (so that this high concentration of sperm will not be diluted by the latter part of the ejaculate).

Retrograde ejaculation, sometimes affecting diabetics, causes sperm to travel backward into the bladder instead of out through the tip of the penis. Certain drugs, such as the blood pressure drug guanethidine, can also cause this problem. Treatment for this disorder used to be incredibly complicated. The man was required to empty his bladder and have it rinsed out. Then, when he ejaculated into the bladder, the sperm was collected and introduced into his wife's cervix or uterus through insemination. Now the condition is often treated by medicines. Ephedrine, Dimetane, or cold tablets such as Ornade may be prescribed to temporarily close the sphincter leading to the bladder.

At one point, freezing sperm was heralded as a possible cure for men with low sperm counts. The logic was that a man could have several ejaculates of his semen, collected over a period of days or weeks, frozen together. Once numerous deposits had been made, they could be defrosted and the wife inseminated with the aggregate semen, which was assumed to contain many times more sperm than a single ejaculate. Unfortunately, while freezing the sperm of a fertile man seems to have little effect on that sperm's fertilizing ability, many of the sperm of infertile men die off in the freezing process, so this technique has been pretty much rejected.

• *LOOKING TOWARD NEW CONCEPTIONS*

Also rejected as a "treatment" for male or female infertility is adoption. The myth used to be that the couple who adopted a child would relax, stop worrying about their infertility, and achieve a pregnancy. This was actually a cruel misconception on the part of some doctors and friends of infertile couples. A number of large-scale studies of infertile couples found comparable spontaneous pregnancy rates among those who adopt and those who do not adopt.

Despite increased research, the tests and treatments described in this chapter cannot always keep pace with the many hazards to fertility in our modern life.

"Thirty years ago, our success rate for treating infertile couples was 55 percent," notes Dr. William G. Karow, director of the Southern California Fertility Institute. "Even with all the advances, the rate is still 55 percent. While we are now able to do a much better job treating ovulatory problems in women (with drugs like Clomid and Pergonal), we have not got an adequate solution for dealing with the huge increase in infections and tubal disease."

If you are an infertile couple, you should first try to achieve a pregnancy by the use of treatments described in this chapter. Ken and Janet Robertson, for example, were able to have a baby in the traditional manner after finally tracking down and treating the cause of their infertility. But for those of you who are not able to conceive with a boost from infertility specialists, it is time to start thinking about the New Conceptions—creating a child through such processes as *in vitro* fertilization, artificial insemination, or surrogate mothering.

4 ❧ The Role of Genetics

A basic understanding of genetics is important for all parents-to-be. It is especially important if you and your spouse might be carriers of a potentially serious genetic disorder or are an infertile couple who want to know more about the genetic traits of sperm donor, surrogate mother, egg donor, or embryo donor. A midwestern couple who are planning to use a surrogate put their concern this way: "We know that environment and heredity interact in shaping a child," explains the wife. "And even if heredity only has a fifty percent influence," adds the husband, "we'd like to have some control over that fifty percent."

For today's potential parents, genetic testing and counseling are a form of crystal ball gazing that was unavailable to their own parents. It was not until the 1950s that the nature and number of chromosomes (the chains of genes) were identified and isolated as the blueprint for a human being.

As scientists investigate more and more closely, they have learned that many birth defects, as well as diseases affecting people late in life, can be traced to the genes that a person received from his or her parents. Genetics research and infertility research are intimately related in at least four ways. Genetic testing can be used to diagnose certain types of infertility. It can be used during pregnancy to tell a previously infertile couple whether their long-awaited child is free from particular genetic disorders. It can help an infertile couple choose an appropriate sperm donor or surrogate. Genetics is also a reason that an individual decides to be "infertile" by choice, foregoing conceiving a child of his or her own because of the risk of passing on a serious defect.

The keys to heredity are the chromosomes and the genes. Most cells in your body have forty-six chromosomes—twenty-three from your mother, twenty-three from your father. The reproductive cells, the egg and sperm, however, in their mature stages have only twenty-three chromosomes, a combination of those from the mother and the father.

The chromosomes are made up of chains of hundreds of genes. Since there are two sets of chromosomes, there are two sets of each type of gene; these are known as gene pairs.

When a child is conceived, an egg with twenty-three chromosomes is fertilized by a sperm with twenty-three chromosomes from the man. Of the genes in each pair, one is from the mother and one is from the father.

Two of the chromosomes are known as the sex chromosomes. A normal female has two X sex chromosomes, while a male has one X and one Y. When you conceive a child, the egg provides an X chromosome, but the sperm may bear an X or a Y, since the father could pass on either. Once the egg is fertilized, it divides over and over again until the fetus has the trillions of cells necessary to make up its entire body. Because all the cells originated from that original fertilized egg, they all have identical chromosomes. As the fetus develops, its cells begin to perform different tasks. Ultimately, it will have two hundred different cell types in its body—each with the same chromosomes.

The workers in these industrial cells are the genes. "Each gene in the chromosome is a coded message that produces a single protein," explains Dr. Zsolt Harsanyi, a geneticist who, with Richard Hutton, wrote *Genetic Prophecy: Beyond the Double Helix.* "The proteins assemble to take part in the creation of blue eyes, bones, nerves, organs, and muscles and work to keep the body running smoothly."

Not everything always moves smoothly in this process, though. Sometimes the child will inherit a genetic defect and a gene pair will not produce the right protein or a group of gene pairs will go awry in their work.

With as complicated a task as creating a normal human being, there are many ways the gene pairs can err. These problems in the process, causing the genes to produce the wrong protein, are known as genetic defects. We all have approximately four to ten genetic defects. "In all humility," avers biologist Dr. Bentley Glass, professor emeritus at the State University of New York at Stony Brook, "I know of at least three obvious ones I possess."

Sometimes your own genetic defects do not affect your life but could be hazardous to your children. Some defects have a range of ways in which they can manifest themselves. A defect that affects you mildly, causing, for example, poor eyesight, could affect your child tremendously (resulting, for instance, in blindness). "This happens when the genetic defect is modified by other genes or by external circumstances, such as an illness or an accident that upsets normal controls and precipitates the injury," explains Glass.

Dr. Zsolt Harsanyi has summed up the genetic component of reproduction as follows: "As we reproduce we play a genetic dice game, with the odds enormously in our favor, but with potentially harmful consequences for our children if we should lose."

• GENETIC DEFECTS

There are basically four major types of genetic defects—chromosomal abnormalities, polygenic defects, single gene defects, and X-linked defects. Any of these difficulties can occur in a number of ways: the parent could have been born with the defect and passed it on to the child through the sperm or egg; the parent could have been born without the defect but developed it due to excessive exposure to drugs or radiation or other hazardous substances and then passed it on to the child; the parent could be free of the defect, but a biological error in transmitting the genetic information to the embryo could have caused the problem; or errors could have occurred as the embryo's cells divided.

A *chromosomal abnormality* occurs when the child has the wrong number or wrong type of chromosomes. The most well-known chromosomal abnormality is Down's syndrome, in which the infant has an extra copy of chromosome number 21.

"One out of every two hundred babies has an abnormal chromosomal construction, of which about half will suffer severe physical problems," reports Dr. Philip Reilly, a Boston City Hospital

physician, lawyer, and author of *Genetics, Law, and Social Policy.*
Chromosomal errors affect many areas of bodily function since the
initial error is present at conception and is repeated in each of the
millions of cells in the growing embryo. Older mothers are at
higher risk for having children with abnormal chromosomes.
About 1.5 percent of the children born to women over the age of
thirty-four have an unusual chromosome pattern. Older men also
have a greater likelihood than young men of fathering a child with
a chromosomal abnormality. In fact, in one quarter of the children
with Down's syndrome the extra chromosome comes from the father, not the mother.

Usually testing the parents gives no hint of the disorder. The
problem generally does not appear in the parents' chromosomes
but is caused by an error in the process of passing the chromosomes on to the children.

A second type of problem is a *polygenic disorder,* involving a
faulty interaction of two or more genes on the chromosomes. If
the fault is in the genes that are responsible for the child's mouth,
the child may have a cleft palate. Polygenic disorders of varying
severity affect up to two of every one hundred children born.

In a polygenic disorder, several genetic defects are occurring at
the same time. "An analogy is the occurrence of a car accident due
to the combination of a slippery road, twilight, heavy traffic, worn
brakes, and a sleepy driver," wrote Dr. Jurgen Hermann and Dr.
John M. Opitz in a medical journal. "No single factor would have
been sufficient to cause the accident."

The third problem is the *single gene disorder,* caused by a defect
in a particular gene pair. These disorders are of two types—dominant or recessive. There are currently nearly fifteen hundred diseases that are thought to be dominant single-gene disorders. They
include achondroplasia (a type of dwarfism), some forms of chronic
glaucoma (which causes blindness), Huntington's chorea (which
causes degeneration of the nervous system), and hypercholesterole-
mia (a high level of cholesterol in the blood that may lead to heart
disease). With a dominant disorder, the parent who carries the
gene is also at least somewhat affected with the disease. The affected parent has one normal gene and one faulty gene in the spe-

cific pair causing the disease, but because the defective gene is dominant, the normal gene cannot compensate for the problems caused in the faulty gene.

Since the child inherits only one of the two genes in a pair from each parent, there is a fifty-fifty chance that the gene that parent passes on to the child will be a faulty one and the child, too, will suffer from the dominant genetic disorder. Sometimes, though, the problem will not manifest itself at birth but will appear much later in the child's life. Huntington's chorea, for example, does not generally appear until the affected person is in his or her late thirties.

In the case of a recessive disorder, the person who has one faulty gene in a pair is not affected by the disease. If you have a recessive disorder, you might not even notice the defect because the normal gene in the pair will successfully complete all work assigned to the pair.

Since carriers of a faulty recessive gene are healthy themselves, they might marry each other without realizing they both carry the same harmful gene. Suppose you marry a person who has a defective gene in the same pair that you do. Since your child will inherit one gene from the pair from each parent, he or she may end up with your defective gene and your spouse's defective gene and the pair might not be able to perform their critical function.

If you and your spouse each had one normal gene and one gene for the disease in a given pair, the potential for having a healthy child would depend on which gene your child inherited from each of you. Since each child's gene pairs contain one gene from each parent, the child potentially could get two faulty genes (one from each parent), one faulty gene from the mother and one normal one from the father (or vice versa), or two normal genes. That child's chance in the gamble is quite good—the child will be affected with the disease only if he or she receives two faulty genes, a one in four chance.

There are about eleven hundred single-gene recessive disorders, including sickle cell disease (a blood disorder that primarily affects blacks), cystic fibrosis (a disorder affecting the muscles and sweat glands), phenylketonuria, also known as PKU (a deficiency in an essential liver enzyme), galactosemia (an inability to metabolize milk sugar), thalassemia (a blood disorder that primarily affects people of Mediterranean ancestry), and Tay-Sachs disease (a disorder of the nervous system that affects mostly Eastern European Jews).

The idea of a recessive disorder is confusing to many people. When they learn they have a single gene for sickle cell or Tay-Sachs, they worry that they themselves will become ill and suffer. But those with a single gene for a recessive disorder (known as carriers of the trait for the disorder) are healthy. It is only the person who inherits two such genes (not a carrier but an affected individual) who actually suffers from the disorder.

X-linked disorders, the fourth type of genetic difficulty, affect males who inherit the defects from their mothers. In this situation, the defective genes occur only on the X chromosome. These defects are generally recessive. Since every woman has two X chromosomes, there is a 50 percent chance she will pass on her defective X to her children and a 50 percent chance she will pass on her healthy X.

The daughter of a woman with an X-linked disorder is generally unaffected. Because she gets an X from her mother and an X from her father, even if she gets the unhealthy X from her mother, its defects are made up for by the healthy X her father gives her. Since a son always gets a Y from his father, an unhealthy X from his mother will *not* be compensated for and he will suffer from the disease.

Over one hundred X-linked disorders are known. Hemophilia (also known as bleeding disease) is the most well-known X-linked disorder. It affects one in fifteen hundred children and is treated by infusions of clotting factor from the plasma of healthy people.

Duchenne's disease, a form of muscular dystrophy, is another X-linked disorder. Although it affects only about 1 in 100,000 children born, the effect is devastating. An affected boy seems normal at birth, but his muscles soon begin to deteriorate. By age ten, he is in a wheelchair. He will probably die by age twenty.

New research has disclosed that a certain form of mental retardation in boys is caused by another X-linked disorder, known as Fragile X. "Couples are definite candidates for testing for this disorder if they have a family history of mental retardation, especially in males," observes Myrna Ben-Yishay, a genetic counselor at the Albert Einstein College of Medicine in New York. "There is a test that can be performed through amniocentesis for Fragile X, but most couples are not aware that it can be offered to them."

• FIGURING THE ODDS

If both you and your husband are carriers of a recessive disorder, your child has a one in four chance (that is, a 25 percent chance) of being affected with the disorder. This does not mean that if the parents have one affected child, the next three children will be healthy. Rather, like a true game of chance, *every child* of the couple has a 25 percent chance of inheriting two faulty genes and being affected with the disorder.

At the annual meeting of the American Fertility Society in 1982 in Las Vegas, Dr. Mitchell Golbus, a genetics expert in the Department of Obstetrics and Gynecology at the University of California, San Francisco, explained the concept: "The dice do not know how they came up last time. The same is true in reproduction. I don't care what the last nineteen kids are. There is still a one in four chance."

Likewise, if you have a gene for a dominant disorder, there is a 50 percent chance that each child you have will inherit the gene and suffer from the disorder. If the mother carries an X-linked disease, there is also a 50 percent chance that her sons will get it. If you have one affected child, that does not mean that the next one will be healthy. It is like flipping a coin each time to determine whether heads or tails (affected or not affected) will come up. As geneticists point out, "Chance has no memory."

• NEW FRONTIERS IN GENETICS

Although the field of medical genetics is advancing rapidly, there are still many things that scientists do not know about the 100,000 genes in a human body. They do not know what causes some genes to switch on during a particular phase of life or turn off during another. They have not yet identified exactly what bodily part or function each gene is responsible for. So far, they can only say definitely what about one thousand genes actually do. With the zeal of a conquistador setting out to explore the New World, these geneticists are racing to solve the riddle of the body's blueprint.

One new line of research may revolutionize the types of genetic predictions that can be made about people. This research scrutinizes the proteins that are made by the genes of chromosome number six in each human cell. These proteins, human leukocyte antigens (HLAs), are found on the surface of the cell. Each person has ten antigens, five inherited from each parent, of a possible ninety-two or more different types.

"There they function as an important part of the body's identification system, a set of highly visible ID cards," remarks Zsolt Harsanyi. They are almost as unique as fingerprints. "Mathematically, there are a couple of hundred million combinations. It is highly unlikely that any one person on earth is identical in his or her HLA type to more than a dozen or so people," Harsanyi explains.

The interest in antigens came about when doctors first began to perform organ transplants. They learned that the more similar the HLA types between the donor and the recipient were, the more likely the transplant would be successful. Since HLAs are like ID cards, the body's disease-fighting system will attack cells with an HLA different from its own.

The interest in HLAs does not end with its application to transplants. Research begun a decade ago has now found tentative evidence that people with certain antigens are more likely to get certain diseases. Harsanyi elaborates on how this works.

"People who become ill ask, 'Why me?' In recent years, we have learned that the secret as to why one person becomes ill while another, subjected to the same environment, stays healthy is partly contained in the genes. Now, researchers have found associations between gene products and disease. For example, people with the antigen B 18 are more likely to get high blood pressure than people without that antigen."

As more information is uncovered about HLAs, HLA screening

might take its place next to genetic screening as a basis for a couple to decide whether they should try to conceive together, whether they should continue a pregnancy, or whether they should choose a particular sperm donor, egg donor, or surrogate.

• *WHERE TO GO FOR GENETIC INFORMATION*

If you are interested in information about genetics, there are a number of places you can contact. In addition to asking questions of your obstetrician or gynecologist, you can seek advice from a professional who specializes in genetic counseling. That person may be a physician with advanced training in medical genetics or perhaps a person who is not a physician but has a degree in genetic counseling. If you would like to know of a genetic counselor or genetic testing center near you, call your local March of Dimes or write to the March of Dimes Birth Defects Foundation, 1275 Mamaroneck Avenue, White Plains, New York 10605; or the National Genetics Foundation, 555 West 57th Street, New York, New York 10019.

Often your own doctor is not the best person to turn to when you want genetic information. The field is changing so rapidly— the genetic bases for fifty to one hundred or more illnesses are discovered each year—that a doctor who is not a genetics specialist may not be totally current. In fact, one quarter of the medical schools do not even offer courses in genetics. In addition, according to Philip Reilly, "effective counseling may require many hours, suggesting that physicians are not the best providers." You might instead seek out a genetic counselor or a medical genetics clinic that has a team of professionals who specialize in evaluation and counseling.

• *WHAT GENETIC EVALUATION ENTAILS*

Zsolt Harsanyi speaks of "genetic prophecy," by which physicians and scientists can predict certain defects and susceptibilities an individual or his or her potential child might have. The data upon which they make those predictions come from many sources—the biological parents' family histories, the results of laboratory tests, and studies of the incidence of disease among similar couples.

The evaluation by a medical geneticist is based on information gained from a variety of investigations. To determine whether there is a genetic reason that you are infertile, the geneticist will ask for a family medical history of you and your blood relatives. If the history raises suspicions of a genetic disorder, the geneticist may ask for a blood sample in order to directly visualize your chromosomes under a high-power microscope. This is known as karyotyping. If the geneticist suspects that the problem is with particular genes, he or she will order biochemical assays, tests to determine whether the genes are producing the appropriate products. Such assays may be done from blood samples, urine samples, or skin samples.

The same types of evaluations—family history, karyotyping, and biochemical assays—can determine whether you are the carrier of a genetic defect that you might pass on to the child. Similarly, the tests could be used on a sperm donor or surrogate mother to help ensure that he or she does not pass on a serious genetic malady to your child.

Once a pregnancy is under way (whether achieved naturally or through one of the New Conceptions), additional tests are available to predict whether that particular fetus has a serious disorder. Since certain of the child's gene products leak into the pregnant woman's bloodstream, some blood tests performed on the woman can provide information about the fetus' health.

Ultrasound is also available to detect certain physical abnormalities of the fetus while it is *in utero*. During this painless procedure, sound waves are bounced off the pregnant woman's abdomen to give a picture of the fetus on a special screen.

An even more definitive genetic test, performed between the thirteenth and fifteenth week after conception, is amniocentesis. Amniocentesis is done by inserting a needle through the mother's abdominal wall and withdrawing amniotic fluid from the womb. No anesthesia is required. Although some doctors use novocaine on the spot where the needle will be inserted, others do not. Doctors do an ultrasound scan so that they can determine exactly where the fetus is before the needle is inserted.

The fluid that is withdrawn is then grown in a special culture and tested for chromosome abnormalities and abnormal levels of chemicals that indicate a genetic defect.

The results of the tests are obtained within three weeks. Among other things, the chormosome test reveals the sex of the fetus.

Since the results of amniocentesis are not received until between the sixteenth and eighteenth week of pregnancy, a woman who decides to abort based on those results requires a second trimester abortion. On the horizon is an alternative technique for diagnosing fetal defects known as transcervical aspiration (TCA), which could be used as early as six weeks after conception. With TCA, the physician uses ultrasound as his guide to pass a tube through the cervix to the point of the trophoblast (that part of the embryonic sac that will become the placenta). A few fetal trophoblast cells are removed through suction and subsequently analyzed for chromosomal abnormalities and certain genetic defects.

Countries like Italy and France are leading the way in transcervical aspiration to analyze trophoblast cells. The impetus has been their large Catholic and Muslim populations, for whom abortions once the pregnancy shows are unacceptable because the community knows. The technique has also been used successfully at University College Hospital in London and U.S. trials are being planned at the University of California at San Francisco.

• THE FAMILY BACKGROUND

To make the most out of genetic screening, you should start thinking about genetics and your family's health history well in advance of the meeting. If you include a self-addressed stamped envelope with your request, the March of Dimes will send you a helpful booklet explaining genetic testing and a worksheet on which you can plot the medical backgrounds of yourself, your spouse, and various relatives. (Write to March of Dimes Birth Defects Foundation, 1275 Mamaroneck Avenue, White Plains, New York 10605.) This will allow you to gather, in advance of the counseling session, information such as whether parents, grandparents, or other relatives had high blood pressure, paralysis, mental retardation, or other diseases—all questions that a counselor will ask.

Of particular importance is information about any relatives who died in childhood. Since the connection between genes and disease was discovered only recently, the victims of genetic defects who died in past generations may not have been viewed as having a genetic problem. They may have been labeled as having died of pneumonia, convulsions, or "failure to thrive." "However, an accurate diagnosis can sometimes be made in retrospect in the counseling session," comments Dr. Laurence E. Karp, Director of Obstetrics and Gynecology and Reproductive Genetics at the Swedish Hospital Medical Center, Seattle, and author of *Genetic Engineering: Threat or Promise?*, and predictions can then be made about whether the disease may strike your children.

Even old photographs can aid a genetic counselor in determining the risks for your children. Karp recounts a case where a deaf child was brought to the Medical Genetics Clinic at the University of Washington. The child's parents wanted to know if there was a genetic basis for the child's deafness and, if so, the risk of subsequent children being deaf as well.

The clinic geneticists decided that the child might have Waardenburg syndrome, a genetic form of deafness that is caused by a dominant single gene. If it was a dominant gene, one of the parents, as well as some of that parent's ancestors, should be suffering from the disease.

The geneticists searched for the symptoms of the syndrome—deafness, white patches of hair, light swatches of skin—in the parents. Both seemed completely healthy. The mother did have a small, light area of skin on her back, but this was not enough to make a diagnosis that her side of the family had the dominant gene for Waardenburg syndrome. The diagnostic team was at a loss. Then the mother remembered that her long-dead grandfather was terribly hard of hearing.

"A hastily unearthed sepiatone print of a family reunion showed that the old man had sported a tremendous white forelock," relates Karp. "This was evidence that Waardenburg syndrome did run in the mother's family. So the couple could be told that the risk of Waardenburg syndrome in their subsequent children would be fifty percent."

From information about you, your spouse, and your respective relatives, the geneticist can construct a pedigree. "This genealogical architecture is of the utmost importance," Karp declares. "Several genetic diseases, most notably some of those affecting the nervous system, have more than one mode of inheritance. By revealing the numbers and relationships of affected individuals in a particular family, the pedigree often defines the correct inheritance mechanisms and therefore the recurrence risks."

Even the parents' ages will figure in the pedigree, since some chromosomal abnormalities (such as Down's syndrome) are more common in the offspring of older mothers or older fathers. Ethnic group is important as well, since certain diseases are more common among particular groups. Eastern European Jews are at a higher risk for Tay-Sachs disease, Greeks for thalassemia (Mediterranean anemia), and blacks for sickle cell anemia.

The pedigree sets the stage for a closer examination of the couple. A doctor can then undertake a physical exam of the couple and subject them to laboratory testing (karyotyping or biochemical assays). These tests help determine the genetic defects the parents have and the risk to a potential child.

• PRE-CONCEPTION GENETIC SCREENING

Genetic screening is important to couples who are having difficulty conceiving and suspect there may be a genetic cause. It is also critical for couples who may be at risk of passing on a genetic defect to the child.

GENETIC SCREENING TO DIAGNOSE INFERTILITY

A particular genetic makeup is sometimes the cause of total sterility. Such is the case with Turner's syndrome, in which a woman is born with a single X chromosome in each cell rather than the normal two X's. The woman suffering from this rare and uncorrectable malady is born without ovaries. Another chromosomal abnormality causing sterility is Klinefelter's syndrome, in which a man has an extra X chromosome, so that his karyotype (the complement of chromosomes) is XXY rather than XY. Although he probably looks normal, he usually will have small testicles and azoospermia, a total lack of sperm.

Although artificial insemination by donor (AID) has been available for decades to couples who cannot conceive due to the husband's chromosomally caused sterility, until recently there was no alternative other than adoption for the couple in which the woman had Turner's syndrome. Now, however, they can turn to a surrogate mother. In an even more stunning advance, one doctor has reported achieving a pregnancy in a woman with Turner's syndrome by implanting a donated embryo. Since a woman with this chromosomal abnormality produces no eggs, she cannot contribute the genetic material to a conception. However, if properly stimulated with hormones, she can carry a donated embryo in her uterus. Thus the alternatives of embryo transfer, embryo adoption, or artificial embryonation, discussed in detail in Chapter Nine, are now open to her.

In contrast to these chromosomal abnormalities, the connection between the person's genetic background and infertility may be more subtle, resulting not in sterility but in difficulty in conceiving or maintaining a pregnancy.

"Genetics plays a role in common gynecological disorders such as endometriosis or polycystic ovarian disease," notes genetics expert Dr. Joe Leigh Simpson, professor of obstetrics and gynecology at Chicago's Northwestern University School of Medicine. Even if the exact link between the gene and the problem is unknown, Simpson believes that if there is evidence of genetic endometriosis in a woman, the doctor should consider contacting sisters or other female relatives to warn them that they might develop endometriosis as well. The sisters could be advised not to delay childbearing and that they should use oral contraceptives rather than the IUD so that endometriosis does not thwart their own childbearing plans.

For the woman who suffers miscarriages, preventing her from carrying a baby to term, genetic testing may lead to an explanation of why these miscarriages are occurring.

"When your mother or my mother had a spontaneous abortion," Simpson points out, "they thought it was due to falling down the stairs. Now we know that at least half of the miscarriages are due to genetic causes." About 15 percent of all recognized pregnancies terminate in spontaneous abortions. Nearly half of the abortions in the first trimester are due to a genetic defect in the child. Generally, it will be possible to conceive again and have a normal child. If you repeatedly miscarry, however, you should have genetic studies performed on your blood to determine whether there is a chromosomal basis for the abortions. About 7 percent of repeat aborters do have a chromosomal problem.

Recent exciting research in infertility has linked some types of spontaneous abortions to human leukocyte antigens (HLAs). Doctors have found that if the mother and father have similar types of HLAs, the pregnancy has a higher than normal chance of aborting, usually around the twelfth week.

A July 11, 1981, article in the British medical journal *Lancet* revealed that couples with similar HLA types who are prone to miscarriage can now be treated. Doctors Colin Taylor and W. Page Faulk treated three women, each of whom had had three previous miscarriages, yet had normal reproductive organs and no hormonal disorders. By giving each woman transfusions of blood from people with a blood type different from that of her husband, the doctors were able to introduce different HLAs into the woman's body. All three gave birth to healthy babies.

Not only should the mother and father be tested to try to pinpoint the cause of repeated miscarriages, but also, medical front-runners advocate, the aborted fetus should be tested as well. At a medical conference, Dr. Bryan Hall, associate director of the Birth Defects Clinic of the University of California at San Francisco, surprised the audience of obstetricians by recommending that they send *every* miscarried or stillborn fetus to a laboratory for testing to determine what went wrong and how it could be prevented in the next pregnancy.

One obstetrician in the audience said he had never considered doing that: "I just tell the parents, 'Nature has made a mistake. It's a blessing.'" Hall compared that approach to practicing medicine in the Dark Ages. "We can't just sweep this under the rug," he maintained. "We should get full-body X rays of the fetus, karyotypes, tests on skin or lung tissues. All the San Francisco hospitals do this. They have found that half the aborted fetuses were physically abnormal, and forty to fifty percent of those were chromosomally abnormal. This helps provide a diagnosis so that we can advise the family about the next pregnancy."

FERTILE COUPLES AND PRE-CONCEPTION SCREENING

As recent advances in genetics have allowed doctors to make specific predictions about a couple's ability to have a healthy child, many gynecologists and obstetricians have begun to offer genetic information and testing to parents-to-be or refer them to specialists in medical genetics. "Every couple should have some degree of surveillance to see if they are at increased risk for passing on certain genetic disorders," advocates Joe Leigh Simpson. "At the very least, a couple should seek genetic counseling if either of them has a disease with a genetic component or has produced an affected offspring or if the mother is over thirty-five and therefore more likely to have a child with chromosomal abnormalities." In addition, he points out that certain ethnic groups may be at higher risk for certain genetic diseases.

Some couples who have given up on the possibility of having children together are not infertile in the traditional sense. They are physically capable of conceiving, but they have decided against pregnancy for fear that they will pass on some dread hereditary disease or illness.

As more maladies are traced to genetic roots, couples face tough decisions about whether they want to bring an affected child into the world. Some will take the risk of having an unhealthy child, others will decide to adopt children, while still others will use the new reproductive technologies to bear a child who is biologically related to one of the couple.

Milton and Cheryl Golden (not their real names) face just that sort of decision. They are of Eastern European Jewish origin and had read in a magazine that people of their descent are more likely than other individuals to be carriers of Tay-Sachs disease.

Since Tay-Sachs is a recessive gene defect, a person with the Tay-Sachs trait is completely healthy. But if *two* people with the Tay-Sachs trait marry and have a child together, there is a one in four chance that the infant will have Tay-Sachs disease. The disease is a crippler, a killer—a heartbreak for the parents and a nightmare for the child. A child diagnosed as having Tay-Sachs disease will suffer from blindness, convulsions, an inability to feed orally, and other physical deformities. His or her life expectancy will be four years. The medical costs for care during that brief life span will be about $35,000.

The Goldens went to their doctor for a blood test and learned they were carriers of the trait. It was the most traumatic moment of their four-year marriage, for they both knew that they could have had healthy children if they had married someone else, someone who was not a carrier. But they have decided to stay together, and the questions they now face are enormous.

Since there is only a 25 percent chance that their child will be affected, the Goldens must decide whether they will go ahead with pregnancy anyway, attempting to beat the odds. If they can live with the choice of abortion, they might choose pregnancy and have amniocentesis to determine whether the child is affected with Tay-Sachs.

The Goldens are still in the process of making their decisions. If they do not feel they could abort an affected child, yet feel it would be unfair to take even a chance of inflicting such suffering on a child, they may turn to one of the new reproductive technologies. Since there is no chance that Milton or Cheryl would have a child with Tay-Sachs if he or she were having the child with someone who did not have the Tay-Sachs gene, they could have one child with Cheryl receiving artificial insemination with the sperm of a donor who is not a carrier and another by using Milton's sperm to fertilize a noncarrier surrogate mother. That way, instead of having one child who is genetically all theirs they will have two children who are each half theirs.

If you knew that any child you conceived had a 50 percent chance of being stricken with Huntington's chorea, which causes a person's nervous system to degenerate late in life, would you take the risk of getting pregnant? If you learned that the fetus growing within you had an HLA type that predisposed him or her to a grave illness, would you continue the pregnancy?

Those couples who think their risk of bearing a child with a serious genetic defect is too high may take advantage of one of the

New Conceptions, such as the use of artificial insemination or a surrogate. These options have already been used by parents with chromosomal, polygenic, dominant gene, and recessive gene defects, ranging from diabetes to Tay-Sachs. Because genetic research is still in its early stages, some couples have opted for a new reproductive technology even though they are unsure about whether their own problem is genetic. Karen Deerfield (not her real name) suffered a serious birth defect that affected her bladder and urinary tract but could not be told conclusively whether the cause was genetic. Her desire not to see her child suffer as she has is leading her to attempt artificial embryonation, a procedure discussed in Chapter Nine.

Karen's husband's sperm will be used, through artificial insemination, to fertilize an egg in a woman's body. After fertilization, the egg will be flushed out and implanted in Karen's body. Thus, since the child will not have any of Karen's genes, there will be no chance she could pass her problem to her child.

GENETIC SCREENING AND THE NEW CONCEPTIONS

Even a brief introduction to genetics underscores the importance for those using a new reproductive technology to choose their donors carefully. A sperm donor, egg donor, or surrogate mother (womb donor) could pass on a serious genetic defect to your child. It is therefore important to request that the doctor take a careful family history of the donor and perform a karyotype or biochemical assay if it appears that the donor may possibly be the carrier of a defect.

Denise and Paul Luigi (not their real names) learned too late about the need for genetic screening when you choose a new reproductive technology. The couple had tried unsuccessfully for five years to have a child. The problem, they finally learned, was with Paul. His semen samples showed only a few sperm, all dead or inactive. He was thirty-one and she was twenty-nine when they turned to artificial insemination by donor (AID), through which sperm of an anonymous fertile male was injected into Denise's cervix to achieve a pregnancy.

Denise became pregnant with the second insemination. The

child was a girl, Jean, who was bright and active for about the first six months of her life. Then her health began to deteriorate. When she was fourteen months old she stopped speaking and lost coordination. A few months later, she lost the ability to crawl or sit. Then she began to have seizures. The diagnosis: a disease similar to Tay-Sachs. The anonymous donor, her biological father, had apparently been a carrier.

An article in the *New England Journal of Medicine* by Dr. William Johnson discussed Jean's case and stressed the need for genetic screening of the donors of sperm to ensure that their sperm does not unwittingly unleash a genetic disease on the long-awaited child. "There is no reason why this type of problem should not occur again or become more frequent as the use of such insemination increases," wrote Johnson. "Thus, it is possible that some families who use artificial insemination to overcome infertility will have children with genetic disease." Even if you and your husband might not have had a genetic problem if you had a child together, genetic screening of the sperm donor, egg donor, or surrogate is advisable.

In addition to an evaluation of the donor's family history and possible genetic testing, you will want to get a list of various medical problems that the donor's relatives have had.

Although the exact genetic mechanisms have not been uncovered yet, it is known that certain diseases—strokes, heart attacks, specific cancers—run in families. Illnesses encountered by your genetic relatives may be likely to strike you. That is why when you see a new doctor or enter a hospital, they ask you about the diseases that have afflicted your various relatives. It is important for your child to have such a history. If your child was born through the use of AID, for example, you will not want a doctor to assume that the child will have the same maladies as your husband and his relatives do. Instead, you might want the doctor to be on the alert for any signs of the illnesses the donor's relatives had.

Geneticists predict that genetic profiles will become an important tool in the future to help people decide about what type of job to take, which foods and environments to stay clear of, and whom to choose as a mate. To ensure that the child you create through a new reproductive technology does not go through life ignorant of his or her genetic past, it is important for you to learn as much as possible about the donor. You might even want the donor to fill out one of the March of Dimes family history worksheets discussed earlier.

• GENETIC TESTS AFTER CONCEPTION

Genetic testing on potential parents produces information about the likelihood that any child they conceived would suffer from a given genetic disease. In the past decade, however, additional genetic tests have been introduced to diagnose whether a particular child that the mother is carrying suffers from the defect.

Genetic screening during pregnancy can be important for a couple who, after many years of infertility treatments, finally conceive. For years, that couple may have been saying, "I would give anything for a child"—while what they generally mean is, "We would give anything for a *healthy, normal* baby." After many disheartening years of trying to achieve pregnancy, most couples are not prepared for the further devastation of having a child with cystic fibrosis or a youngster with Tay-Sachs disease who would die before his or her fourth birthday.

Couples who have been infertile and then achieve a pregnancy are often slightly older than those couples who are able to get pregnant as soon as they start trying. This increased age makes the couple inherently more likely to have a child with certain chromosomal disorders, such as Down's syndrome. Nearly 4,000 of the 3.4 million babies born each year in the United States suffer from this malady. A child born with Down's syndrome has widely spaced eyes, a short, stocky build, and, frequently, heart malformation and profound retardation. The possibility of having a child with Down's syndrome increases with the mother's age, especially once the mother reaches her mid-thirties. "On the average, one baby with Down's syndrome occurs in every twenty-five hundred born to eighteen-year-old mothers but one out of every fifty babies born to women over age forty-five have this disorder—a fiftyfold increase!" warns Philip Reilly.

The tests that can be done during pregnancy to learn more

about the health of the child include blood tests and amniocentesis. Some previously infertile couples who finally get pregnant undergo these tests. Couples who use a surrogate mother often provide in their contracts that the surrogate must undergo such testing.

The one blood test that is widely used during pregnancy is a test for alpha-fetoprotein. It is used as a preliminary step in diagnosing a fetus affected by a neural tube defect. Such a disorder can cause encephaly (where part of the brain is missing, causing stillbirth or death shortly after birth) or spina bifida (where the spinal cord protudes through the backbone, potentially causing paralysis of the legs, loss of bladder and bowel control, and, sometimes, mental retardation).

Any mother could give birth to a child with a neural tube defect. The disorder affects nearly two out of every one thousand pregnancies in the United States and, unlike Tay-Sachs or sickle cell anemia, is likely to strike children of any race or ethnic group. Unlike Down's syndrome, the age of the mother does not matter.

The neural tube defects are polygenic disorders, caused not just by one gene but by an unknown combination of a number of genes. Because an interaction of various types of genes causes the problem, there is no known test that can be done on a couple to determine whether their child is likely to have a neural tube defect. The only tests are those that are done while the pregnancy is under way.

Less than a decade ago, scientists discovered that the opening caused by the neural tube defect leaks a high amount of alpha-fetoprotein (AFP) from the fetus into the amniotic fluid and into the mother's bloodstream. Now a simple test with blood taken from a pregnant woman can determine whether the AFP level is elevated. The test costs about twenty dollars.

Even if a couple believes in abortion, they would be making a terrible mistake if they decided to abort a child merely on the basis of a blood test showing a high AFP level, for there are other reasons for a high reading. The level of AFP increases as the fetus ages, so a high AFP level might indicate that the pregnancy is farther along than the couple thought. The woman could be carrying twins, which naturally would elevate the AFP level to twice as much. "In fact, the *least likely* reason for an elevated AFP level on a blood test is a neural tube defect," asserts Dr. James Macri, director of the Neural Tube Defects Program at the State University of New York at Stony Brook.

A blood test alone, then, will not give a definitive diagnosis of a neural tube defect. The pregnant woman with an elevated AFP should next undergo ultrasound. This scan may pick up a healthy sign, such as the fact that a woman is carrying twins, or further confirm a neural tube defect, such as a fetus with an abnormally shaped head characteristic of anencephaly.

If the ultrasound reveals no explanation for the AFP, the woman can undergo amniocentesis. If there is a high level of AFP in the amniotic fluid, this is convincing evidence that the child is affected by a neural tube defect.

With each type of test, more women find that their fetus is unaffected. About fifty women in one thousand will have an elevated AFP in a blood test, but after ultrasound and amniocentesis, forty-eight of the fifty will learn that their babies do *not* have a neural tube defect.

Amniocentesis, a technique for testing the fetus for genetic defects while it is still in the uterus, is used to diagnose about one hundred other genetic maladies as well. In 1975, the federal government put its stamp of approval on amniocentesis, since a four-year study of the procedure on two thousand women supported by the National Institute of Child Health and Human Development had judged the technique to be safe and accurate.

"Deciding to undergo amniocentesis was hard," reports Joan Liebmann-Smith, a research sociologist at the Center for the Study of Women at the City University of New York Graduate Center. "I had an infertility problem and I knew if I lost the child due to the process I would probably never get pregnant again. I wasn't sure whether I would be able to go through an abortion of this long-awaited child. The genetic counselor we consulted said she was happy she had children before amniocentesis was available. These are tough decisions to make."

"I found amniocentesis to be emotionally painful and medically painless," recounts Lynn Drew, a clinical social worker who became pregnant at age thirty-nine after seven years of surgery, medicines, and other infertility treatments. The pregnancy was almost as important to the infertility specialist as it was to Lynn; he came with her and held her hand while another doctor performed the test.

Amniocentesis is an enormous breakthrough in prenatal diagnosis. Before it was available, definitive prenatal diagnosis of certain genetic defects could be accomplished only by ever so carefully trying to reach the squirming fetus in the uterus and to take a sample of its blood. This was a hazardous procedure that killed 5 to 10 percent of the fetuses tested.

Amniocentesis is much less dangerous. A study of three thousand amniocenteses performed in San Francisco found a 1.5 percent risk of spontaneous abortion after amniocentesis. It is not clear whether the amniocentesis itself caused the miscarriage, though, since 1.2 percent of the patients who had made appointments for amniocentesis miscarried in the week *before* the appointments (before they even had the procedure). Recent studies estimate that one in two hundred fetuses is at risk of harm from amniocentesis.

Couples should consider amniocentesis if the woman is over age thirty-five, if they are members of an ethnic group that is susceptible to certain genetic defects, or if their histories reveal a genetic defect in the family. It is estimated that as many as 400,000 pregnant women annually should have amniocentesis. About 3,000 had it done in 1974; now the figure is estimated at 15,000 to 20,000.

Amniocentesis, like other forms of genetic testing, is not done as a matter of course. Although 95 percent of nine hundred women surveyed in 1979 by *McCalls* magazine felt that at-risk couples should have genetic testing, not all doctors inform couples of the availability of genetic tests for themselves and amniocentesis for their offspring. In fact, a study by Dr. Sara C. Finley and her husband Dr. Wayne H. Finley of women undergoing amniocentesis at the University of Alabama revealed that more than 40 percent of the women had heard of amniocentesis from television, newspapers, and magazines rather than from their doctors.

Often it is only the well-off or well-educated couples who find out about and request amniocentesis. In the San Francisco study, 56.2 percent of the mothers undergoing amniocentesis and 78.6 percent of their mates had attended college. The average income of the people seeking amniocentesis was $25,271.

The information acquired from amniocentesis is almost always reassuring. In a 1977 study of ten thousand women undergoing amniocentesis, 97 percent were found not to have the defect being tested for.

"Amniocentesis itself need not be scary," says one geneticist. "It's safe, easy and merely provides information from which to make choices. Those choices may be difficult, but most people are reassured that the baby is okay and they can stop worrying for the rest of the pregnancy."

• *MAKING THE MOST OF GENETIC INFORMATION*

A couple who have undergone genetic testing or otherwise sought genetic counseling are understandably apprehensive. They are about to learn information that will affect their future lives—their concept of themselves, their dreams of having a family. Often they have recently suffered the loss of a pregnancy or of a child due to a wrenching genetic disease and they wonder what their chances are of bearing another such child. According to Dr. Henry Lynch, chairman of the Department of Preventive Medicine and Public Health at the Creighton University School of Medicine in Omaha, Nebraska, the couple who visit a genetic counselor are not as caught up initially in the genetic problems as they are in the "guilt, anxiety, apprehension, and fear."

To make the most of the information gained through genetic evaluation, it is crucial that you understand everything that the genetic counselor discusses with you. A follow-up study done at Johns Hopkins School of Medicine of clients of genetic counselors found that one half of the people did not understand enough to be able to make appropriate decisions based on the information. If you do not understand something the counselor is saying, ask to have it explained further or in a different way. Bring paper to take notes at the meeting for future reference.

One emotionally difficult aspect of genetic counseling is finding out that the genetic defect has been passed on from one parent only (as in the case of the deaf boy Karp mentioned who inherited his malady from the mother's side of the family). Some doctors do not disclose whether a defect is inherited from the mother or from the father because they believe this will be a source of marital friction.

If you want to achieve parenthood, however, it is important to know how the genetic defect is passed on. If the husband has the problem, the wife will be able to have a healthy baby with AID. If the woman carries a defective dominant gene or a sex-linked disorder, the couple might consider using artificial embryonation or a surrogate mother. If both partners are carriers of a recessive gene disorder, either partner could have a healthy child by a noncarrier. The risk occurs when both partners create a child together, since that child might get a double dose of the defective gene.

In such a case, you and your husband might want to have two children, each biologically related to one of you (for example, one by AID and one by a surrogate). Thus, it is important to find out which of you has a particular genetic defect—not so that you can lay blame, but so that you can determine what means you should choose to have a child who is biologically related to one of you.

The information you will be getting at the counseling session is complicated, so it may be a little difficult to take it all in at once. Try to have the counselor send you a follow-up letter detailing what was expressed in the session. Some genetics services routinely send these follow-up letters. This has helped to increase couples' understanding (to 76 percent rather than the 50 percent the Johns Hopkins University study found). It also gives couples a permanent record to refer to or show relatives who might be similarly at risk of having children with a genetic defect.

While you should learn as much as possible at the session, it is important to remember that the point of the counseling is to get information, not make an on-the-spot decision regarding whether you should have children or continue a current pregnancy. Studies have found that many genetic counselors are influenced by their own personal feelings about how they would deal with a child who has a particular defect—and thus may go beyond providing information and try to persuade a family according to their own criteria. Yet a counselor's focus on, for example, the economic cost of raising a child with a certain malady may not match the couple's own concerns. The couple may prefer to make their decision based on whether an affected child will nonetheless have the ability to love and be loved. "Research has found that, even at an unconscious level," says Reilly, "counselors may be pressuring patients to make a certain decision."

In addition, counselors have a divided allegiance. On the one hand, they are supposed to respect the personal choices of the couple. On the other hand, the medical geneticist may be trying to reduce the number of children born with serious diseases, and thus may try to discourage a couple from having a child even when there is a fifty-fifty chance or more the couple would have a healthy child.

Sometimes the way a counselor expresses the risks reveals his or her leaning. For example, Karp notes the difference between saying that there is a 4 percent risk the child will have a certain defect and saying there is a 96 percent risk that he or she will not, even though they mean the same thing. Often, clarification of risks is necessary to cut through the counselor's biases.

"It's terrifying to hear, after you give birth to a child with a cleft palate, that your chance of having another affected child is forty times more than the general population," Karp points out. "It's different when you think of the risk as only four in one hundred, since the general population risk is one in one thousand."

Although counselors should be neutral in their discussion of your options, "failure to press for one course of action or another is unusual in medical practice and may be a difficult course for many doctors to follow," admits Dr. Barton Childs, professor of pediatrics at Johns Hopkins University School of Medicine. He analyzed the medical journal articles written about genetic counseling and found that a number of doctors and genetic counselors seek to prevent genetic defects by pressuring parents who might possbily pass on such a defect to forego childbearing.

The American Medical Association Judicial Council in June

1983 cautioned doctors doing genetic counseling and screening that they should "avoid the imposition of their personal moral values and the substitution of their own moral judgment for that of the prospective parents. The ethical and moral decisions have to be made by the family and should not be imposed by the physician."

Once you have obtained the factual information from a genetic counselor—such as what the odds are that you will have a child with a certain genetic disease—the tough decision-making begins. At home, you and your spouse will have to face many important questions. If you are at the pre-conception stage, will you try to get pregnant or is the risk so high and the potential genetic disease so devastating that you will take advantage of one or more of the New Conceptions? If you (or your surrogate) is already pregnant and learn that the fetus is affected by a genetic disorder, will you choose abortion or not? What will life be like for a child with the disease and what will your life and that of your other children be like if you do give birth to an affected child?

In the course of reaching a decision, read everything you can about how the genetic disease will affect your child. With Tay-Sachs, it is fairly clear that an affected child will die early in life after suffering paralysis, respiratory difficulties, and other extreme problems. In a number of other diseases, however, the grave picture being painted by some genetic counselors is in dispute. A special clinic at Children's Memorial Hospital in Chicago has found that a high percentage of those children born with spina bifida, for example, can lead a normal life once adjustments are made for physical disabilities.

At some point in the pre-conception stage, though, you will have collected sufficient information to know whether your future child could be at risk for a genetic defect and how serious that defect will be. Then the decision whether to conceive becomes intensely personal. "Some couples will consider a one in four risk of bearing a child with cystic fibrosis to be unacceptably high," comments Reilly, while "others will perceive that it is three to one in their favor."

Whether couples will try to have children when they are at risk for passing on a harmful trait depends on the severity of the defect and the magnitude of the possibility it will occur. In an English study of 421 couples, 54 percent of the couples who had a 10 percent or greater risk of having a child with a genetic defect stopped having children. When the risk was less than 10 percent, only 30 percent of the couples stopped having children.

If you are making a decision during pregnancy, you may want to abort. When 2,187 women underwent amniocentesis in a 1974 study by the National Foundation March of Dimes, sixty-two of the fetuses (3 percent) had a serious genetic disorder. All but two of the mothers with seriously affected fetuses chose abortion.

If your decision is to continue the pregnancy and give birth to the child, you should investigate whether there is any special treatment or equipment the infant will need to aid his or her development. Kent Smith of the Spina Bifida Association of America suggests, for example, that infants with spina bifida be delivered in a neonatal center equipped for high-risk deliveries. His group is compiling a list of such centers across the country.

Some couples panic when they hear the term genetic defect associated with their child. One woman reportedly opted for an abortion when she was told she had a one in twenty chance of giving birth to a child with a genetic defect of a harelip—which is purely a cosmetic disorder.

If you find out through amniocentesis or transcervical aspiration that your fetus has a genetic defect, learn more about the type of life an affected child would have, and your ability to care for an affected child. If you have had several pregnancies and have aborted them due to genetic defects, it may be time to think about one of the new means of reproduction.

• *GENETIC DISCRIMINATION*

It cannot be stressed enough that whether you are using genetic testing and counseling before conception or amniocentesis and counseling during pregnancy it is crucial for you to find out what potential effect a genetic defect will actually have on your child.

Even the scientific community has been wrong about the problems caused by certain genes and chromosomal abnormalities.

Take the case of the XYY syndrome. In most male babies, the mother contributes an X chromosome and the father a Y chromosome. In some rare cases—an estimated one out of nine hundred—*two* Y's fertilize the mother's X egg. This extra Y can be detected by testing done either during amniocentesis or after the child is born. Since the extra Y causes no physical defect that would affect the person's functioning, XYY males initially attracted little attention. Then, around 1965, Scottish and Danish researchers found a greater proportion of prisoners with the XYY chromosome complement than in the population at large. This led to speculation that the XYY was a "criminal gene," causing its bearer to be tall, violent, and mentally slow.

Since then, the XYY myth has been debunked. Studies have shown that there are around 200,000 American males with the XYY chromosomal complement, the great majority of whom have no criminal tendencies. "In fact, further research indicates XYY's in prison may actually be *less* aggressive than their XY counterparts," claims Harsanyi.

The confusion between carriers of a recessive single gene disorder and those affected by the disease has also led to genetic discrimination.

One out of every ten American blacks has the sickle cell trait, a single gene for sickle cell anemia. The gene does not affect their own health, but if two carriers of the gene marry, there is a one in four chance that their child will inherit the sickle cell gene from each of them and have sickle cell anemia. Such a child will have certain abnormally shaped red blood cells that do not move as readily through the blood vessels as their normal counterparts and that do not transport oxygen as efficiently.

When widespread screening for sickle cell trait began in the 1970s, many people did not realize that people with the trait—a single gene—did not have the disease. As a result, some insurance companies raised their rates for blacks who were carriers but were not themselves affected by the disorder. In addition, the Job Corps advised blacks with the single gene to choose undemanding work, counseling them to choose electronics assembly, for example, rather than carpentry or automobile body repair. It took a massive educational campaign by concerned doctors and scientists to correct the misimpression that sickle cell carriers were unhealthy themselves.

• DOCTORS, GENETICS, AND THE LAW

Amazing strides have been made in genetics solely within our life span. In many areas of science, it would take decades for the information to filter out of the laboratories to the general population. But in the area of genetic testing an unusual turn of events is now forcing doctors to bone up on genetics and get the word out to their patients. Doctors are finding out what happens if they do not tell couples that they might produce a child with a genetic defect— and offer them tests to find out whether they are genetically at risk. If they do not explain and the couple goes on to conceive an affected child, their next meeting with the couple may be in a courtroom. Couple after couple have brought suit against doctors who did not explain genetic risks or who incorrectly performed genetic tests. These lawsuits seek to make the *doctors* financially liable for certain costs related to rearing the child. Similar lawsuits might be possible if a doctor carelessly arranged for you to use a semen donor or surrogate mother who carried a serious genetic defect.

After Hetty Park's first child died of polycystic kidney disease, a fatal hereditary disease, she wanted another child. Before getting pregnant, though, she asked her doctor what the chances were that her next child would be similarly afflicted. He erroneously declared that it would not happen again. Park got pregnant and gave birth to a second child with polycystic kidney disease, who lived only five hours.

Around the same time, thirty-seven-year-old Dolores Becker found out that she was pregnant. Her doctor did not tell her that her age increased the risk of giving birth to a child with Down's syndrome. Nor did he recommend amniocentesis to test the fetus. Nine months later she gave birth to a Down's syndrome infant. Both she and Hetty Park sued their doctors. In an action for "wrongful birth," they argued that they had wanted children, but children without birth defects. They blamed the defects on the physician for not counseling them adequately about genetics.

The highest New York court heard both cases. The court decided that the Parks and Beckers could recover from the doctors the cost of the care and treatment of the affected children until their deaths. In the case of a Down's syndrome child, such costs can be enormous—$250,000 or more. A judge who disagreed with the decision was horrified at the results of the case, claiming they created a "medical paternity suit."

An even more novel legal tactic was initiated by Hyam and Phillis Curlender. As descendents of Eastern European Jews, they knew that they were at increased risk for having a child with Tay-Sachs. They asked their doctor to test them for the disease and were joyous when the results came back negative. They achieved a pregnancy soon after, resulting in the birth of a girl, Shauna Tamar Curlender. Shortly after the baby's birth, though, it became clear that something was wrong. Shauna was sluggish, could not focus her eyes on objects, and was unable to sit up or hold her head up. The laboratory results had been misread. Shauna would soon suffer blindness, convulsions, and the other effects of Tay-Sachs disease.

In the summer of 1980, a California court heard a lawsuit on Shauna's behalf. The infant Shauna (through her father Hyam Curlender) was suing the laboratory that had erroneously informed her parents that they were not Tay-Sachs carriers. Shauna's suit against the laboratory claimed, in essence, that she had a right to be born healthy or not to be born at all.

Other infants in the past had tried to make such claims for "wrongful life" but they had never won their cases. In 1979, for example, the Pennsylvania Superior Court rejected such a case, stating, "Whether it is better to have never been born at all rather than to have been born with serious mental defects is a mystery more properly left to the philosophers and theologians, a mystery which would lead us into the field of metaphysics, beyond the realm of our understanding or ability to solve."

The California court reversed the trend. The court ruled in Shauna's favor, saying it would be unfair to her if the justice system "retreated into meditation on the mysteries of life" rather than taking an objective view of the child's pain and suffering.

While courts are beginning to show more sympathy for the couples who give birth to a seriously ill child due to physicians' negligence, some legislatures are lending protection to the physicians. Laws recently enacted in Minnesota, South Dakota, and Utah, for example, prohibit lawsuits charging wrongful birth or wrongful life.

The cases for wrongful life and wrongful birth sent shock waves through the obstetrics community. "As recently as five to ten years ago, people didn't think of bringing such actions," notes Dr. Jeffrey Shane, an obstetrician and attorney who heads the Division of Medical Legal Consultation at the Armed Forces Institute of Pathology. Doctors are now pressured to provide sufficient genetic information so that couples can choose whether the wife should become pregnant in the first place and, if she is already pregnant, whether she should abort the affected fetus. To be able to make the best use of this information, you should become familiar with the types of genetic screening available for a couple and the types available for the fetus. You should also understand what will take place in the genetic counseling session and what limits exist to the predictive powers of medical genetics.

• *THE EMOTIONAL FACTOR*

A National Academy of Sciences report points out that genetic screening differs radically from nongenetic screening (such as medical testing to learn whether you have an infection) and that emotional problems result from this difference. According to the Committee for the Study of Inborn Errors of Metabolism of the National Research Council of the National Academy of Sciences, "nongenetic screening is usually intended to discover people with diseases due to influences outside themselves and for which they may feel no responsibility. But genetic screening discovers something within a person's own makeup that may threaten his self-esteem or cause him to feel guilty of transmitting some 'blight' to his children."

Couples who have given birth to a child with a genetic disorder—or who are at risk for such a child—often feel that they are being punished for something bad they have done.

For some couples, the general counseling session announcing the results of their tests or an amniocentesis may be their first realization that they might never have a healthy child. After that emotional blow, one or both may find that they could have a normal baby if only they were married to someone else.

"If their baby's condition is due to a recessive gene, then it means each of them could have a normal baby with almost anyone else," observes genetic counselor Myrna Ben-Yishay of the Albert Einstein College of Medicine in New York City. "That kind of situation can really rock a marriage. It's a difficult test."

Some couples do not survive the test. Marriages crumble at the stress of the guilt and despair. One English study seemed to provide some hope for the emotions of couples who undergo genetic testing and counseling. It found that divorces among such couples three to ten years later were no higher than that of other comparably aged Britains. A closer look at the statistics, however, showed that, among those who found out that they had a genetic defect and decided not to have children as a result, the divorce rate was three times the British average.

Of particular trauma is the X-linked disorder. "If the condition is recessive, as with Tay-Sachs or sickle cell, a mutual support system can develop since both carry the same gene which is not working correctly" comments Ben-Yishay. "With an X-linked disorder, there are much greater emotional upheavals, since the gene is passed on through the woman. She may feel a lack of self-esteem since she is not able to provide her husband with normal, healthy males."

The woman can be helped to overcome this trauma if her husband is supportive and persuades her that he did not just marry her for children, but for her other fine qualities. One husband comforted his wife by explaining, "It doesn't matter to me that we have this problem. I wouldn't want any other woman to have my children."

The testing itself may cause an emotional trauma. People formerly accepted the birth of an unhealthy child as God's will, but now parents are faced with making choices about whether a child will be conceived, or whether a developing fetus will live or die. Many couples are unprepared for the responsibility.

At the time amniocentesis takes place, the fetus is already in at least its thirteenth week of development, complete with tiny limbs, face, and heartbeat. Perhaps there already was a baby shower, or a room made ready, or a name chosen. When the results of that test come back, the couple may feel a close bond to their "child," so that the prospect of abortion is particularly painful to them.

Unlike most abortions, which are for women who had not intended to get pregnant, the couple in this situation *wants* a child. Another contrast is that an unwanted pregnancy is usually ended before the woman begins to "show." An abortion for genetic reasons ends a pregnancy that friends and relatives know about, if for no other reason than the size of the pregnant woman's abdomen.

A study of thirteen families who aborted for genetic reasons found a high rate of postabortion depression among the couples. Nevertheless, 77 percent of the people said they would opt for amniocentesis and, if necessary, abortion in a future pregnancy. In some instances, health care personnel can increase the sadness. One woman in the study was a carrier of hemophilia B, which has a 50 percent chance of affecting each son. When she and her husband learned through amniocentesis that the fetus was male, they chose an abortion because there was no test to show whether the child would actually be affected. The woman's postabortion depression was deepened by a nurse who commented, "You would have had such a beautiful boy."

Anne and Joe Barbera had one healthy child, Bridget, when they aborted what would have been their second child because tests indicated that the child had spina bifida. The abortion, painful for Anne because the pregnancy was far along, was especially tough on Bridget, who had been excited about the idea of having a new baby in the house.

"We had shared the pregnancy with Bridget from the beginning because we didn't want her to be jealous," Anne explains. "I would even take her to the doctor's appointments with me. When

I found out something was wrong, though, I didn't know how to tell her. After the abortion, I said the baby was sick and went to heaven. Because I was so upset, Bridget became upset, too. She would have nightmares. Whenever we'd see a pregnant woman, she'd say, 'Is that baby going to die and go to heaven?'"

Later, when Anne became pregnant again, she quit her job, stopped seeing anyone socially, and told no one except her parents, Joe's parents, and one close friend. She did not want to have to face other acquaintances if she aborted again. For this child, the amniocentesis revealed no abnormalities and Bridget finally got the sister she wanted.

Couples who have amniocentesis wonder about its emotional effect not only on their close families (including any children they might have), but also on the child they decide to have after testing. Will their child—healthy or not—feel less special knowing that the parents had undergone amniocentesis? Will the parents, who might have been prepared to abort if the amniocentesis showed any problems, feel strangely about the child once it is born, as if it had been expendable?

In one family in which a woman aborted a fetus with a genetic defect, she came home to find her other child hiding in a closet, refusing to come out. He was afraid his mother would try to get rid of him, too.

It will be a few years before the children of amniocentesis are old enough for their psychological reaction to the procedure and that of their siblings can be fully investigated. But there have been some studies of the parents who have undergone it. Episcopal priest John Fletcher, a bioethicist at the Clinical Center of the National Institutes of Health, has done research in this area. He feels that "considerable moral suffering was involved in making the decision to request amniocentesis. Wanting children desperately, yet having to contemplate the possible abortion of a defective fetus, these parents were often torn asunder with worry."

However, Fletcher found that couples who underwent amniocentesis felt closer to their tested children. Some felt that they had known their tested children longer than they had known their untested children.

"One could speculate that prenatal genetic information can

deepen the sense of intimacy between parent and child as it hastens and increases the assumption of parenthood before birth," notes Fletcher.

Not all genetic testing conveys happy news. The couple may learn that their child-to-be will have a hopeless affliction. They may also find out that, like couples subject to infertility, there is no one they can really talk to about it. "Other family members may not be supportive," warns Ben-Yishay. "They may disapprove of genetic testing, saying, 'It's not in our hands, it's in God's hands.' Or they may find the topic complicated to understand and not understand the seriousness of the couple's concern.

"Some couples will not acknowledge a pregnancy to themselves or friends or relatives until after they have had the amniocentesis," Ben-Yishay continues. "They want to avoid having to explain that they had the test and they chose an abortion."

Anne Barbera feels it is important to let people know of the existence of tests to pinpoint spina bifida and anencephaly in a fetus. "One woman I know miscarried a spina bifida child at seven months," says Barbera. "She hadn't even known the child had spina bifida. Where was her doctor? Was he asleep? What could he have been thinking of that he didn't offer her the test?"

Since not all doctors inform their patients about genetic counseling, Barbera has taken it upon herself to spread the word, even when it means dealing with harsh criticism. "When people ask you how could you have murdered your child, there's really nothing you can say," explains Barbera. "I'm a Catholic and I always said I would *never* have an abortion. I criticized other people. Now I've learned you cannot predict what you will do until you are in that situation. I did what was best for me and my family."

Some couples are afraid to disclose the genetic defect to anyone for fear it shows that they are inferior. It does not. We all have between four and ten genetic defects. Moreover, some genetic "defects" have both a good and a bad side to them. A gene that causes a subceptibility to one disease may cause a heightened resistance to another. The sickle cell gene causes a blood disease in blacks in America but is beneficial to blacks in Africa since it protects them against malaria.

Sometimes, the couples do not even want members of their

families to know about the diagnosis. Genetic counselors then confront tough ethical questions. Information that a medical professional learns about a patient is confidential. But what if a counselor learns that a woman carries a gene for hemophilia? Should the counselor have the right or responsibility to tell the woman's sister that she, too, may be a carrier?

Most relatives in that situation would want to know that they were at risk for bearing an affected child. In a study of the relatives who were contacted and told (with the original couple's permission) that they may carry a harmful gene, over 90 percent appreciated receiving the information. Some genetic counselors even advocate counseling sessions with relatives present.

• THE SOCIAL REACTION

The couple who makes childbearing choices based on genetic reasons is subject not only to their own emotional reaction and that of close relatives but also to that of society at large. There are those who feel it is terribly wrong to abort a genetically defective child or even choose to use a sperm or egg donor to avoid the possibility of giving birth to a child with a particular genetic defect.

The Roman Catholic Church opposes amniocentesis. In addition, right-to-life groups oppose the process because they believe it invariably leads to abortions. Mitchell Golbus, however, foresees a time when parents will be able to treat, rather than abort, a fetus with a genetic defect. Already, laser surgery has successfully eliminated fetal tumors while the child is still in the uterus. Golbus himself performed an impressive operation in which he placed shunts in the kidney of a child in the womb.

For some opponents of genetic screening, it is not the possibility of abortion but the concept of eugenics that is troubling. Their resistance to the use of genetic prophecy today is due to historic movements in the past, such as that of Hitler's Germany, that claimed "genetics" as their basis for sterilizing or killing people thought to be undesirable.

Even in America, where we cherish our individual freedoms, groups have made attempts to create a better race. "The period from approximately 1900 to the 1930s witnessed the growth of the American Eugenics Movement as an attempt to improve humanity by altering its genetic composition through encouragement of breeding among those presumed to have desirable genes (positive eugenics) and discouragement of breeding among those presumed to have undesirable genes (negative eugenics)," commented Morris B. Fiddler, of the Department of Pediatrics at Northwestern University Medical School, and Children's Memorial Hospital, Chicago, at a University of Illinois workshop on Frontiers in Genetics.

As part of that movement, thirty states tried to legislate "worthiness" for childbearing by passing laws to sterilize people who were thought to be alcoholic, feeble-minded, or to possess criminal tendencies. These laws remained in the books until the 1970s, when most were repealed.

In addition to these pseudoscientific attempts to eliminate negative traits in the gene pool, attempts to create a better race have added to the scorn surrounding much of genetics. The California sperm bank that offers semen from Nobel Prize winners is such an attempt. Its founder, Robert Klark Graham, sees the sperm bank as a way to improve the American gene pool by creating more intelligent children.

Even a rudimentary knowledge of genetics uncovers flaws in Graham's approach. Intelligence is not a single gene trait but is the result of the interaction of a number of genes and the effect of the environment as well. For that reason, there is no guarantee that a child born of a Nobelists's sperm would grow up smart. In addition, since the possibility of certain genetic defects increases as the donor's age increases (especially over age sixty), the children born through Graham's program via sperm of older Nobel Prize winners may be at risk for genetic diseases.

If you are having genetic testing done on yourselves or a donor, it is important to realize the limits, not just the benefits, of such testing. It will tell you the chances that your child will suffer from a particular, serious, genetic defect. It will *not* allow you to choose a superchild with the eye color, I.Q., and other traits you want.

Perhaps it is just as well that genetic research has not progressed that far. Parents in the 1980s already have an enormous responsibility and control based on the limited genetic information they have now and the few decisions (to conceive or not; to abort or not) that they must make based on that information. If any test would allow them to choose special traits, it would truly seem that they were playing God.

Besides, it would be tremendously difficult for you and your spouse to decide on the traits your child should have (rather than just the serious defects to be avoided).

"You need do no more than go to a P.T.A. meeting to discover that some people want their children to be highly competitive, while others place a major premium on noncompetitiveness," writes Karp in his book *Genetic Engineering: Threat or Promise?* "Some parents hope for children with great athletic skills, others desire that their offspring excel at school, and still others feel that their children will be best off as gentle, kind and unselfish mediocrities."

Karp has qualms about the children of presumed "superior" AID donors (and a similar concern could be voiced about the children of extraspecial surrogates or egg or embryo donors).

"How would they interact with their "inferior" legal fathers? Would relative 'superiority' of one's biological father become a new status symbol? What of the child whose donor-father fell from favor? Alas for Young Stalin in Russia and Young Nixon in America!"

"In my personal opinion this situation differs radically from ordinary artificial insemination where the biological father is unknown and the couple accept the child as their own," reflects pediatrician Robert Golenboch of Danbury, Connecticut. "Here, the couple may feel less like parents and more like the caretakers of a famous man's baby.

"And think of the enormous pressure on the child," he continues. "Everyone will be waiting around for the first time $E = mc^2$ comes out of his mouth."

Moreover, the traits you would choose for your child might not be the ones he or she wants. "The skinny boy whose mother insists on violin lessons may wonder whether he might not have been big like the other boys if his mother hadn't traded size for musical talent before he was old enough to be asked what he preferred," Harvard professor Thomas C. Schelling told a symposium of scientists meeting to discuss "Genetics, Man and Society."

In addition, sociologist Amitai Etzioni points out that even if couples did get their wish about their child's genetic traits, they could be disillusioned. "The shoppers who ask for high I.Q. genes may be quite disappointed when they find they have a clever but unmotivated, or smart-alecky, child, or one who misapplied his or her talents, or looks down on his 'dumb' parents."

• *WHAT GENETIC TESTING CAN DO*

Genetic testing is not at the point where it will let you pick, Chinese-menu style, the traits of your children. At the present time, the science of genetics can tell you only if your child-to-be will suffer from particular genetic defects. Even if testing on you and your spouse and an amniocentesis-based analysis of the child's cells came back fine, the baby may still be born with a defect or disease. Not all deformities are genetic and even those defects that are genetic cannot all be tested for. Amniocentesis, for example, can investigate only one hundred of the thirty-three hundred known genetically linked diseases.

Despite its present limitations, genetic testing brings new choices and opportunities to childbearing. As more is learned about the inheritance of genetic defects, more people will choose to use donors so as not to play Russian roulette with their children's health. In addition, infertile couples who use donors of sperm or eggs should insist on genetic screening of these individuals.

5 ❦ The Emotions of Infertility and Medical Genetics

Infertility touches all aspects of a couple's life. It climbs into bed with them. It colors how they talk to their parents. It dictates their social schedule—arranging vacation plans so that treatment schedules will not be disrupted, and keeping them away from baby showers or christenings, where their sadness is overwhelming.

"Sex is timed; vacation is timed," states Lynn Drew, a clinical social worker who tried for seven years before she was able to have a child. "It takes a toll in marriage, job, body image, everything. It touches every area of your life. Nothing goes unscathed. Nothing."

"People have fantasies about having a child," says psychologist Aphrodite Clamar. "They feel they'll have a wonderful time, go to bed with a bottle of champagne and get this beautiful baby nine months later. No one enters marriage expecting to hear that they are infertile. People become depressed, unhappy, and wonder, 'What happened to our dream?'"

"The couple that can't have children faces a philosophical crisis," declares psychiatrist E. James Lieberman, associate professor at George Washington University School of Medicine. "They ask themselves, 'What am I here on earth for? What will be left of me when I'm gone?'"

When infertility enters a marriage, plans and dreams get put on hold. The relationship is derailed, the usual activities set aside.

"For years, our life has been in limbo," reports Stella Baer (not her real name). "We have tried in every way to accommodate the birth of a child. We live in a building with an elevator, so I won't have to exert myself walking down stairs if I get pregnant. I don't have a full-time job, so that I won't have to let down an employer if I take to bed to avoid a miscarriage."

Women and men, individually and as couples, undergo an emotional turmoil with infertility that can shatter their basic concepts of themselves. Physicians, especially busy infertility specialists, may be unprepared or unwilling to help the couples work through the intricacies of their emotional maze. Worse yet, the doctors may be oblivious to the way their style of dealing with the couple worsens the trauma.

You and your spouse can, with sensitivity and understanding, work your way through the maze. It will take a level of communication that you may never have achieved before. But the effort will be worth it. "Once you survive the emotional and physical stress of infertility, a strength develops and you feel your marriage can survive anything," claims Joan Liebmann-Smith, a research sociologist at the Center for the Study of Women and Society at the City University of New York Graduate Center. She interviewed thirty-five infertile women for her doctoral thesis and has spoken with hundreds more as a copresident of the New York City Resolve. "Most women I interviewed felt their marriages were better for this and that they discussed things with their husbands that they wouldn't have otherwise."

• *THE WOMAN'S FEELINGS*

Throughout history, women have taken the blame for barren marriages. Even today, when it is clear that the husband is just as likely as his wife to be the cause of their childlessness, it is the woman who is initially viewed as the culprit. She is the one who first goes to the doctor for an infertility workup. She is the one who fields the questions from relatives and in-laws: Why haven't you had a baby yet?

Because of the erroneous notion that the woman was the prime cause of infertility in the couple, research into treatments for male infertility has lagged. As a result, even if the problem is caused by the man, the onus of treatment is often on the woman. If the man has a low sperm count, for example, there is not much modern medicine can offer him. So the wife will be treated in the hopes that she will become superfertile, with her reproductive system compensating for his low count.

"It's harder emotionally on the woman," Liebmann-Smith points out. "She is constantly monitoring her body. It becomes an obsession by necessity almost. Every time she goes to the bathroom she checks to see whether she is bleeding or whether her cervical mucus is ripe."

In addition to having the prime physical responsibility for childbearing, women bear the prime social responsibility as well. As little girls, while their spouses-to-be were off playing soldiers or firemen, they were carefully feeding their dolls and changing imaginary diapers. Almost from birth, they have been raised for the role of mother—while boys were being trained to fit comfortably in a variety of roles.

As a result, when the ability to bear a child is denied a woman, the pillars of her self-image tumble. She feels ugly. She blames herself. One twenty-nine-year-old woman worried that her pursuit of a career "had closed the door to motherhood." Many women who discover they are infertile tell their husbands, "You can divorce me."

Some women say they feel different from others and are sure that their infertility is noticeable. One woman, a fine athlete who belonged to a number of clubs and organizations, dropped out of them when she learned she was infertile. She felt her infertility was actually visible.

Dr. Lawrence Tourkow, a Detroit psychoanalyst, describes a woman who consulted him briefly for therapy while she was in college. She got married, and ten years later she was back in analysis. Infertility had destroyed her self-image. "The work we'd done with her feelings of femininity, her pride," says Tourkow, "it was as if someone had taken a sledgehammer to a statue. It was in pieces."

"A lot of infertile women postpone making career advances," Liebmann-Smith discovered. In her dissertation research, she found that infertile women felt they were not able to focus on their

careers. They did not want to get into a position of major responsibility and then have to slow down to guard a long-awaited pregnancy.

"Infertile female doctors put off opening private practices and
took lower level positions," reports Liebmann-Smith. "One woman
turned down a major job as a sports broadcaster for television. She
didn't feel that her infertility would interfere with her ability to do
the job, but she thought the job might be too high powered if she
got pregnant."

"It's easier to plan around a pregnancy than infertility," observes Boston psychiatrist Miriam Mazor, who counsels infertile
women. "The woman is in job limbo, reluctant to make any move.
She's worried that if she takes a new job, she'll have to take three
months off at the beginning of pregnancy."

Passing up career advancement may lead to resentment, though.
"Often the woman becomes resentful because not only is she not
pregnant but also she is not in a high-powered job either," Liebmann-Smith notes.

One woman gave up teaching school to try to have a child, then
learned that her husband was infertile. She resented him for making her give up her children at school without giving her children
of her own. Her anger did not completely disappear until she
was able to have a child through artificial insemination with donor
semen.

"The job limbo is what most infertile women come to me complaining about," states Mazor. "They say, 'I have nothing to show
for myself.' People ask them, 'How come you're not vice president
of your company already if you don't have a kid?'"

• *THE MAN'S FEELINGS*

Men, too, find their concepts of themselves threatened when they
learn that they are unable to father a child. "Men find it stigmatiz-
ing not to be able to impregnate their wives," explains Liebmann-
Smith. "They feel it is a reflection on their sexuality."

Men grow up with the notion that they will *always* be fertile;
after all, men like Pablo Picasso and others fathered children late

in their sixties. "Men have never had to face the prospect of diminished fertility," remarks Sherman Silber, a St. Louis specialist
in male infertility. They are psychologically unprepared for the denial of fatherhood. Many describe themselves as "shooting
blanks."

"In this macho society, the man may totally deny or disbelieve it
could be his problem," warns Dr. William W. Beck, Jr., associate
professor of obstetrics and gynecology at the University of Pennsylvania. "That's why the couple should come in together for the
first evaluation and the physicians should explain from the start
that there is a substantial chance it could be a male problem."

"When it was my wife's problem," admitted one infertile man,
"I could be wonderfully supportive. But when I learned that I had
a problem as well, my masculinity was threatened. I resisted surgery for months, provoking our first major marriage conflict."

The blow of learning he is infertile can lessen a man's sex drive.
In a survey at Mount Sinai Hospital in Toronto, Canada, of sixteen men who were diagnosed as infertile, eleven experienced a
period of impotence.

There may be no place they feel they can turn with their sadness. Tim told his co-workers he was unable to have a child. They
responded with guffaws and began leaving *Playboy* magazines in
his locker and offering to teach him the facts of life.

"Western society provides emotional support for a woman who
is infertile or sterile; her friends give consolation," writes Dr. Ar-
mand M. Karow of the Xytex Corporation sperm bank in a letter
to the *New England Journal of Medicine.* "But a man who is sterile may find himself the target of ridicule from presumed friends
and even from his family."

The potential for ridicule may lead to elaborate deception. One
man, reluctant to face his infertility, conned his physician by bringing in sperm samples of a fertile friend. In other instances, men
with infertility problems have forced their wives to tell friends it
was the wives' fault!

Worse yet, a man may perversely begin to believe his own de-
ceptions. Liebmann-Smith describes a man who had a very low
sperm count with poor motility and abnormal morphology. Even

though he was the cause of their barren marriage, he put the blame on his wife, ultimately leaving her, insisting, "I want to have children so I'm going to find someone else."

• *THE STAGES OF THE INFERTILITY CRISIS*

Some reactions to infertility are colored by the person's sex, since women are brought up expecting to be mothers and society equates male virility with fertility. Other emotions growing out of infertility are common to both men and women.

When Barbara Eck Menning faced infertility she found that, although she had a degree in Maternal-Child Health and Nursing, she did not understand the feelings she experienced. Menning interviewed many couples who were similarly suffering and realized that an infertile person passes through stages that are similar to those Elizabeth Kübler-Ross has identified as the stages of dying. Over a period of time, the individual first denies his or her infertility, then is enraged by it, becomes guilty, feels grief, and then accepts the inability to bear a child, perhaps choosing to adopt or to try one of the new reproductive technologies.

Infertility counselor Ellen Bresnick and Harvard Medical School clinical professor Melvin Taymor interviewed sixty-two couples who sought counseling for infertility. They found that women were more overtly affected by the infertility crisis than were their husbands but that both spouses experienced some degree of guilt, anger, frustration, and isolation. The problems women focused on were slightly different from those that concerned the men. Women were most upset about the possibility of the ultimate failure of the workup and treatment; men were most concerned about problems in communication (which also concerned women).

Why are the stages of dying so relevant to infertility? Because, say infertile couples, a part of you dies when you cannot give birth to your own child. "It is clearly a loss—a loss of a function of your body, or your genetic heritage, of a pregnancy, the loss of all the fantasies that go along with having a biological child," explains Madeline Gupta, a Washington, D.C., psychiatric nurse-practitioner who runs support groups for infertile couples.

"The loss is similar to that of the loss of a loved one," agrees Betty Orlandino, a social worker who founded Human Relations Counseling, which specializes in the psychological aspects of infertility and the new reproductive technologies. "It *is* the loss of a loved one—indeed, the death of the child who was never conceived."

One infertile man being counseled by Orlandino cried when he realized that he would never have an opportunity to teach "his" son to fish or play ball. Miriam Mazor finds that infertile couples mourn the end of their genetic line. This is particularly acute, she finds, among the children of Holocaust survivors who feel the need to reproduce for themselves and for the sake of relatives who were killed by Nazi brutality.

Since they have to try so hard and plan so furiously in their attempt to conceive, infertile couples may be envious and spiteful of other couples who multiply easily. One otherwise stable professional woman said that her infertility caused her to want to run down pregnant women with a car.

"You hate to watch television because there are all those commercials with babies," recalls Lynn Drew, who is now a counselor for the Chicago Resolve chapter. "You hate holidays because that's a family time. Sadness comes upon you out of nowhere, in huge waves, for no apparent reason. Suddenly you're crying. You feel you are losing your mind."

Despite the great loss associated with infertility, society has no mechanism for acknowledging the loss and coming to terms with it. The parents of a stillborn are comforted by loved ones, while the infertile person is largely ignored. Moreover, the barren individual himself or herself may be uncertain when to mourn. The possibility of more tests or treatments may hold out hope for years, even when none actually exists. "I'd rather have it hopeless than uncertain," claims one man.

"I always ask infertile couples whether this reminds them of anything they've ever had an experience with before and they mention death," Ellen Bresnick notes. "It's the same feeling of helplessness and mourning, but there are no socially acceptable channels for it—because what have you lost except your dreams about your whole future."

The couple also face emotional turmoil as they need to make a decision about what will happen if they can not have children of their own. Will they try to adopt? Will they make use of *in vitro* fertilization or artificial insemination? When will they begin to tell other people about their infertility?

Rarely do a husband and wife approach problems in similar ways. Can't you remember a time when your spouse handled a dispute at work or with friends in a way you thought was inappropriate, or gave up on some activity long before you wanted to? The distinctive personalities of you and your spouse make marriage interesting, but they may clash when the two of you have a shared problem—infertility—and must agree on a way to approach it.

Couples experiencing an infertility crisis, even couples in which both are infertile, cannot assume that both are experiencing the same feelings at the same time. You have to try extra hard to learn about what your spouse is feeling and share with him or her your own feelings.

"You've got to respect that each of you may be at a different position in the infertility crisis," advises Madeline Gupta. "One may still be mourning the loss of a biological child, while the other is thinking, 'Let's close that chapter and move on to AID or adoption.' Everyone's timing for the grief process is different. Classically, one person is in the lead, but he or she shouldn't try to push the other one too much. But the one in the lead can quietly do the footwork for the next step, such as finding out about artificial insemination, so that they have a head start when the other person reaches that stage."

To help infertile couples work through their feelings and grieve for their loss, Barbara Eck Menning wrote *Infertility: A Guide for the Childless Couple* and founded Resolve, a national self-help group of infertile couples. She had been struck by infertile couples' feeling of isolation, even though one in six other couples shared their problem. Menning felt that people needed a place to go to discuss their loss, to discuss the trauma of dealing with a "death" that occurred before life.

The meetings of the forty-three Resolve groups across the country are impressive. There is an educational component, with speakers discussing new treatment methods or describing research or how infertile couples react when they finally become parents. But the bulk of the meeting time is devoted to infertile people discussing what is bothering them about their condition, their medical arrangements, their relationships with family members. The Chicago Resolve chapter recently asked infertile couples to bring their parents to a meeting. The parents poignantly described how it felt to be "nongrandparents" and then generation sat down with generation to discuss how they could ease each other's suffering. Resolve also sponsors support groups for men, women, or couples, run by counselors who have experienced infertility. These groups help people resolve their feelings about their infertility and make choices about how they will proceed with their lives once the infertility has been faced.

Throughout the process, keeping a sense of humor is essential. "Without humor, people would never get through the situation of timed intercourse—having intercourse when you least desire to and withholding affection when you feel most like giving it," comments Gupta, who runs Resolve support groups.

Sometimes the humor comes out only when you are in a support group and people begin to discuss the crazy things they have been told to do to enhance their fertility (such as stand on their head). The funny part is that they have actually done it.

"One woman related that she carried her husband's sperm for AIH to the doctor's office in a baggy in her bra, all the while fearing she'd get into an auto accident and the police would think she was crazy when they asked her what was in the bag," recounts Gupta. "Another couple said they had dinner guests coming in forty minutes when they remembered that that was the night they needed to make love. In a split second they were hopping into bed, knowing they'd have to shower, get dressed, and mix the salad before the guests came. Naturally, the doorbell started ringing before they were done."

To keep people's spirits up when everything seems to be going wrong during the infertility workup, the national Resolve staff printed the following column in their newsletter.

YOU KNOW IT'S GOING TO BE A BAD DAY WHEN . . .
by the Resolve Staff

You know it's going to be a bad day when . . .

1. You put the wrong end of your basal thermometer in your mouth.
2. Your infertility specialist posts the following sign in his office: "We only accept cash for visits and tests. Please pay before leaving."
3. You are taking a semen sample in for analysis and a policeman stops you for speeding and asks what's in the jar.
4. Your new puppy chews up 3 months worth of basal temperature charts.
5. On the day of your A.I.D. insemination the doctor cancels because his wife just had twins.
6. The country where you are adopting a baby has a major military coup and all travel in and out of the country grinds to a halt.
7. The only seat on the bus is beside a very pregnant woman with a cute 2-year-old squirming on what's left of her lap.
8. Your Clomid prescription comes in a child-proof cap.
9. You start dating your reports at work with the day of your menstrual cycle.
10. You see a *60 Minutes* film crew and Dan Rather entering your adoption agency.
11. You go into your crowded neighborhood pharmacy for BBT supplies and the cashier yells to the druggist at the other end of the store, "Where are the basal thermometers and what the hell are they?"
12. Your house guests mistake the 24-hour urine collection in the refrigerator for cider.

13. In the middle of your hysterosalpingogram you hear the radiologist say "Oops."
14. Your adopted child comes home with a biology assignment to plot his/her family tree.
15. Your employer calls you in to discuss your bi-weekly absences for "death of a loved one" for the past year and a half.
16. You go into a drugstore to buy a BBT chart and the pharmacist winks suggestively.

Reprinted with permission of Resolve, Inc.

• *UNDERSTANDING YOUR FEELINGS*

As your feelings about your infertility unfold, there will be a profound effect on your relationship with your spouse. "Infertility makes couples take a harder look at each other," warns Mazor. "They begin to assess the marriage at a stage when other couples are too busy with child care to do so."

Infertile individuals often feel "defective" and need reassurance that they are still loved. The fertile spouses may have to cope with feelings of despair when they realize that they could have had a child if only they had married someone else.

The bed can become a battleground. "Infertility essentially climbs into bed with you each night," acknowledges Janet Robertson (not her real name). "It clearly affects what goes on when you turn out the light. Sex loses its pleasure and begins to seem like just a way to get pregnant."

In Liebmann-Smith's study, virtually all the women reported a destruction of their sex life (only two said their sex life was better, crediting it to having to have sex more often). "Infertility wreaks havoc with the couple's sex life," Liebmann-Smith reports. "Either the man finds he can't perform on schedule or the woman says she can't. The couple begins to have sex around the time of ovulation and avoid it the rest of the month. Some worry that they'll never enjoy sex again."

"We had a very good sexual relationship," one patient explained to Bresnick, "until we realized we had a problem. Then it got horrendous. My body and desires did not always match my temperature chart."

Some infertile couples are so aware that they should be making love around ovulation time that spontaneity dwindles from their sex life. Worse yet, one spouse may virtually attack the other to ensure that they do not miss the most fertile day. Neither fatigue nor anger nor other responsibilities can be an excuse to postpone. Mazor recounts that one woman "raped" her intern husband in the house-staff quarters of a hospital when he was on duty on one of her potentially fertile days; the experience was humiliating for them both."

"Sex is no longer a spontaneous act of love," states Lynn Drew. "It's a lousy homework assignment that is graded by the doctor in a postcoital test or graded by you when you wait to see whether you've gotten pregnant. There is an intrusion into the most private part of your life. Some doctors have you mark down on your temperature charts the days you have sex. Some couples feel they have to lie and mark sex at other times of the month so that the doctors wouldn't think they were fighting."

Drew points out that being a slave to the woman's monthly schedule has other ramifications. "Since you only have a short fertile time each month, every time a new therapy is suggested you wait a month to try it. If the doctor says, 'Why don't we try this in January,' and you've got a vacation planned in January, you cancel it. You don't want to miss a month."

While a fertile person might think a month's postponement would not make any difference, the infertile couple does not want to take a chance of missing *any* cycle. One woman who was undergoing AID in New York panicked when she realized she would be in South America at the time she was ovulating. Rather than skip a month, she arranged to have frozen semen shipped down to her.

• *EMOTIONAL ASPECTS OF GENETIC COUNSELING*

When a person learns that he or she could pass on a serious genetic defect to a child, the emotions experienced are similar to those of an infertile individual. "If the person has already had one child with the disorder," observes Dr. Joe Leigh Simpson, professor of obstetrics and gynecology at Chicago's Northwestern University Medical School, "they go through the same sort of process that a person goes through with bereavement, the stages that Kübler-Ross documented. There may be a denial, and then an anger, a lashing out at anyone whether appropriate or not. There is a guilt that they did something that made the baby not normal. This continues until they come to some resolution about the loss of self-esteem."

The people who decide not to procreate due to a potential genetic problem describe themselves with some of the same terms infertile people do: defective, isolated. They, too, mourn the end of their family's bloodline.

The couple who are childless because they do not want to risk having a child with a genetic defect and the couple who abort a fetus that is diagnosed as having a serious defect have other things in common with the infertile couple. They may also be upset when they see pregnant women or couples with infants.

Two neighbors had babies the same week that Anne Barbera underwent an abortion after amniocentesis revealed the fetus had spina bifida. "I hated them," admits Barbera. "I didn't want to see them. I didn't even visit the children until they were six months old."

Sometimes the emotional anguish of infertility and genetic testing combine. One woman in Liebmann-Smith's study delayed childbearing because she was busy with other areas of life. When she and her husband finally decided they wanted a child, they had difficulty conceiving. When they finally overcame their infertility problem, they conceived a Down's syndrome baby.

"It was a double emotional blow," notes Liebmann-Smith. "The woman blamed herself, feeling that delaying childbearing until her thirties had caused both the infertility and the Down's syndrome."

• *EMOTIONAL ASPECTS OF TESTING AND TREATMENT*

As you progress through the workup and treatment, different emotions flare up at different times. Each new test or therapy brings a new assault to your self-image, a new set of doubts about proceeding that must be resolved.

The initial diagnosis of a problem in procreation triggers the stages that Menning has likened to the stages of mourning. Other parts of the infertility or genetic investigation are also emotionally unsettling, such as the fear that accompanies not knowing exactly what will be done to you.

"One man was terrified about undergoing a testicular biopsy," explains Orlandino. "He mistakenly thought the word 'biopsy' indicated he might have cancer. He worried that they would have to remove the testicle. The episode would have been less traumatic if there had been an explanation of the process and the reason for it."

A lack of understanding of what various treatments entail also can raise fears. Women waiting to be artificially inseminated worry that the procedure may require an incision or may involve having sex with the donor. (In reality, artificial insemination is a simple, painless procedure. The woman assumes the position she would for a pelvic examination and then some semen is squirted into the vagina near her cervix.)

At some point, one spouse will want to try a certain technique while the other does not. After several years of infertility treatments of both him and his wife, one husband still resisted the idea of having his wife artificially inseminated with his sperm. "I want to do it naturally," he insisted. His wife was amazed that he would let some notion of artificiality impede them from exhausting all possible treatments. "How can you even believe we are still doing it naturally after all these pills and operations?" she asked.

Some treatments can cause sadness and resentment. When a woman has developed antibodies to her husband's sperm, the doctor will suggest that the husband use a condom when they make love. If the woman has endometriosis, she will be given a continuous dose of birth control pills to create a pseudopregnancy or pills that cause her body to behave as if it were undergoing menopause. All of these treatments require the couple to practice contraception, usually for at least six months, before they can try to conceive.

This approach is disconcerting. If the woman is over age thirty-five, she may feel there is very little time left for her to become pregnant—her biological clock is ticking away as she approaches actual menopause. Yet in an ironic twist of fate, her husband must use a condom or she must take drugs to treat her infertility that stop her from ovulating altogether. In addition, a pseudopregnancy may cause her to feel nausea and other signs of pregnancy—focusing her mind and emotions on childbearing and worsening the psychological trauma of infertility.

For the couple who undergo genetic testing, the emotional response stems from the fact there is no real treatment. Instead, they are offered the option of aborting the fetus.

Doctors Bruce D. Blumberg, Mitchell S. Golbus, and Karl H. Hanson of the University of California School of Medicine in San Francisco interviewed thirteen families who underwent amniocentesis for detection of a genetic defect and aborted the fetus. "It appears that selective abortion shakes the foundation of self-worth, especially to the extent that self-esteem is predicated by societal and personal values upon the ability to create a normal, healthy family," they concluded in the *American Journal of Obstetrics and Gynecology*. They advise doctors to tell people of the psychological aspects of selective abortion before amniocentesis is undertaken.

The new reproductive technologies, appropriate for couples with infertility or genetic problems, may themselves raise emotional concerns. When the efforts at conception involve only one spouse, the other may feel left out, isolated, useless. The husband and his feelings may be overlooked as the wife undergoes AID; a wife may feel totally superfluous when the husband's sperm is used to inseminate a surrogate. Yet there are ways to involve both spouses, even in the new reproductive technologies. Some doctors let the husband inject the donor sperm into his wife for artificial insemination. Some wives take Lamaze classes with their surrogates and become coaches for delivery; they even get to hold the babies before the surrogates do.

When the individual understands what will happen in the infertility or genetic program and takes an active role in the treatment plan, the emotional trauma is alleviated considerably.

"The greater the patient's understanding of his or her body, of the reasons for certain tests and therapies, the more responsibility he or she may assume in sharing the information with the physician, and the more capable he or she may become in understanding and coping," report Bresnick and Taymor in *Infertility*. "Explanations of tests and treatments help allay fears engendered by misinformation and ignorance. The patient may assume a more active, less helpless role. He or she can begin to feel involved in the treatment rather than its victims."

Taymor believes that knowing more about the tests and treatments can also improve the quality of care you get. "If a doctor orders a test for a certain day," says Taymor, "the patient can say, 'I think that's the wrong day of my cycle for such a test,' In that way, she will be getting better care."

Unfortunately, not all physicians are willing to let the patient become a partner in the medical enterprise. "Some physicians want their patients to go on blind faith," says the president of the Chicago chapter of Resolve. "There are decisions to be made in dealing with infertility: whether drugs or surgery should be used, whether one drug should be used over another. And these are decisions the patient should make."

Doctors treating infertility can actually cause emotional problems rather than solve them. Doctors involved in genetics are usually a little more sensitive to emotional issues since they normally work hand-in-hand with a genetic counselor, a person trained in dealing with the psychological aspects of genetic disease and treatment. In a 1983 study of 38 infertile women conducted by Katherine B. Mann and Thalia Maroulis, one third of the women said they found communication with their physicians to be stress producing.

In Liebmann-Smith's study, doctors were derelict in their communication with infertile women. They did not tell them what the tests were about or give them options, nor did they explain about the side effects of drugs. "Or the doctors didn't tell the women to expect pain when they did an endometrial biopsy, then called her a baby when she cried out," Liebmann-Smith reports.

Some doctors are brusque. Others behave totally inappropriately. "A prominent physician told one woman she should just have an affair," states Liebmann-Smith. "And some doctors take miscarriage lightly, saying 'You could have ten miscarriages before I looked for anything wrong with you.'"

Janet Robertson (not her real name) was told by a psychiatrist that she could not get pregnant because she seemed ambivalent about choosing between career and motherhood. "The psychiatrist said this without finding out whether I'd gone through all the tests," she fumed. Years later Robertson learned that the cause of her infertility was endometriosis, which could be treated.

Doctors sometimes make light of the infertility problem early in the investigation and tell the couple just to relax and try to get pregnant. This makes the couple both angry and more anxious. In addition, there is little evidence that tension causes infertility. One patient told Mazor, "When the doctor suggested I was too neurotic to get pregnant, I blew up. I told him that if he thought I was uptight, he should meet my mother! My grandmother was even worse, and she had eight children. I come from a long line of uptight fertile women."

Emotional anguish is rarely the *cause* of barrenness; rather, it is the infertility that causes the emotional upset. "It is imperative that all those who deal with infertile couples understand their already intense emotional distress and realize the infertility itself, may exacerbate existing biological, emotional or social problems," writes Taymor in *Infertility*. "Emotional trauma and its effects, then, are clearly a part of the entire problem of infertility. The physician should recognize and treat the *total* problem of infertility to minimize the overall emotional devastation."

William Beck, Jr., tells doctors, "There are real psychological needs of infertile couples and if we are unfeeling and insensitive, there will be problems." Beck tries to make doctors more aware of the couples' feelings by pointing out the emotionally charged nature of the investigation. "I don't know whether I could go to a stranger and discuss my sexual habits" he concedes. "Be sensitive to timing," he tells the doctors. "You are putting a strain on couples if you only have office hours in the afternoon and request them to have intercourse at 6:00 A.M. in order to do a postcoital. I've never had intercourse at 6:00 A.M. in my entire life. The psychological impact will be far less if we remember how important caring is. There will be a small amount who will get pregnant just because of that caring."

Among the advice that Taymor gives professionals is that "at all times the therapist should be aware of the psychologically harmful effect of the tests and treatment, and one should be prepared to discontinue these when more harm than good is being produced."

According to Taymor, when a urologist is evaluating the husband and a gynecologist is evaluating the wife, the doctors sometimes create emotional problems by creating a "rivalry" between the spouses. The gynecologist may declare, "It's your husband's fault. He's got a low sperm count," while the urologist will put the blame on the wife's poor cervical mucus or occasionally irregular ovulation.

In an article for *Parents* magazine, David Riley summed up the treatment he and his wife had received from infertility specialists: "The doctors we had been to had shown considerably less feeling for us than our Volvo mechanic shows for our Volvo," wrote Riley. "We don't expect doctors to be psychiatrists; we know the difference. But we do expect doctors to make at least a passing acquaintance with the feelings of the patient, instead of treating him as a time-consuming nuisance."

If you feel you are being emotionally aggravated by your physician there are many things you can do. You can stay on top of your own case by reading about infertility tests and treatments in order to supplement the scant information the physician may be giving you. Also, switch doctors if there seems to be a personality clash. Do not delude yourself into thinking that all good infertility specialists are rude and inconsiderate. A bad bedside manner does not signal good technical skills; in fact, an unwillingness to explain or answer questions may be a clue that a doctor is covering up the gaps in his or her own knowledge.

• *RELIGIOUS CONSIDERATIONS AND THE EMOTIONS OF INFERTILITY*

For couples in certain religous groups, infertility is a double trauma. Not only are their personal goals of childbearing thwarted, but also they cannot fulfill the biblical mandate to "be fruitful and multiply." If their religion expects them to forego birth control and bear children, the couple will have no chance to conceal their infertility problem. If they do not produce a child within the first year of their marriage, their infertility will be obvious to members of that community.

Marsha Sheinfeld, president of the Chicago chapter of Resolve, Inc., and an Orthodox Jewess, wrote movingly in the *Resolve Newsletter* of the dilemmas presented by infertility within her religion. In Orthodox Judaism, there are strict rules governing the timing of intercourse and forbidding intercourse during menstruation and during seven bloodless days thereafter. For infertile couples, the time of abstention may coincide with the time the doctor asks them to have intercourse. If the doctor lacks understanding and advises the couple to cheat on their religious beliefs, wrote Sheinfeld, they are then "forced to choose between their doctor, whom they believe to possess the 'cure,' or their religious conscience."

• *SOCIETY'S REACTION TO INFERTILITY AND GENETIC COUNSELING*

"Infertility and genetic counseling touch all relationships, those with co-workers, friends, relatives, neighbors and others," comments Betty Orlandino. Friends may not understand why you feel so hurt. Old rivalries with siblings may take on new intensities.

"If a sister gets pregnant and you can't, you may feel that you failed your parents," Marsha Sheinfeld points out. "You feel hostile and bitter and can't stand to be with her. If she miscarries, you feel guilty, as if it were the result of your evil thoughts."

If you have chosen not to reveal why you cannot have children, you may face constant wheedling from relatives urging you to have a child. If you already have one child but are having problems conceiving again, that child may beg and plead with you to give him or her a brother or sister. The child may also wonder whether you think he or she is so bad that you do not want another child.

"If you have secondary infertility, you may feel that you are taking out your depression on your child," warns Sheinfeld. "You may think, no wonder I can't have another child, I can't even take care of this one."

Dealing with in-laws can be a special trial. One woman was constantly hounded by her mother-in-law to have a child. She finally got angry enough to blurt out: "Go talk to your son. It's his fault we can't have kids!"

Even if you *do* disclose the problem, that is no guarantee the other person will understand your feelings. Many infertile couples are told, "You don't know how lucky you are!" Friends point out the benefits of not having to worry about birth control or begin to list all the difficulties about child-rearing that you will "fortunately" avoid.

Columnist Erma Bombeck was childless for the first six years of her marriage and then suffered two miscarriages. She feels that friends and relatives are not supportive of infertile people. "They get about as much sympathy as an eighty-three-pound woman who is trying to gain weight," wrote Bombeck.

Everyone suddenly becomes an expert in fertility, telling you to just relax and you will readily conceive. "Well, *we* went to Australia for six months to relax and it *still* didn't work," protests a woman who has been trying to get pregnant for six years.

People will tell you that your infertility is "God's will." When a friend said that to Paul Heiden, Paul advised him to discard his toupee because if God intended, the friend would have hair.

If you are seeking genetic counseling, those close to you may try vehemently to dissuade you from undergoing amniocentesis or aborting a fetus that has a serious genetic abnormality. When, after much soul-searching, Anne and Joe Barbera decided to abort what would have been their second child because of spina bifida, people asked Anne, "How could you have murdered your child?"

To a certain extent, people's unfortunate remarks can be handled by pointing out how ludicrous they are or how bad they make you feel. Sometimes the people who have not lived through infertility or genetic testing just do not understand. Then you need a warm cocoon of understanding to which you can retreat. You and your husband can create that sort of emotional support for each other.

• *ESCAPING THE EMOTIONAL MAZE*

As Liebmann-Smith discovered, coping with the physical and emotional crises of infertility can make a marriage stronger. The same is true when the couple discovers a genetic defect that will influence their childbearing. For the marriage to grow stronger, though, you need to discover your feelings about the situation and talk about them.

Couples from all walks of life suffer deeply when they have problems in procreation. No one is immune to the emotional reaction. People who married young, whose friends all have two or three children and who do not have much else in their lives, are devastated by infertility. So are wealthier professional couples who travel and have good jobs. In fact, this group is often amazed when they find out how much having a child means to them.

While procreation problems stir up the emotions of all involved, people react to the crisis in unique ways. According to Mazor, "much of what people feel and do depends on their characteristic way of dealing with other disappointments and losses in their lives. The go-getters continue to be go-getters and have a hard time knowing when to quit. Those people who generally feel like victims of fate in other areas of their life will probably not approach infertility aggressively enough, will not push hard enough and will keep bungling along with the same doctor."

To work your way through your crisis, ask yourself if you are being realistic in your expectations. One woman was upset that she did not get pregnant the first time she tried making love without contraception; she had been trying to time the birth for June, when the academic year ended.

Also, be realistic about the odds you face. Find out what the chances are of a person with your type of infertility problem conceiving or of an individual with your particular genetic risk giving birth to a healthy child. Be honest with yourself and be honest with each other. One woman felt sorry for her infertile husband. Trying to make him feel better, she lied and told him she had a fertility problem, too. This merely angered him later when he found out the lie had delayed them in their decision to undergo artificial insemination by donor.

Also, find out the physical mechanisms that cause the infertility or genetic problem. One woman, not recognizing the hereditary nature of Down's syndrome, tortured herself with the mistaken notion that strenuous activity had caused her baby to be affected with the disorder. A man who refused to believe he could carry an unhealthy gene denied that he was the father of his affected child.

Lydia (not her real name) erroneously believed that her husband's low sperm count signaled a lack of interest in her. She tried seducing her husband, wearing outlandishly sexy outfits, all the while thinking, "If only I was a more desirable woman, my husband wouldn't have the problem."

The infertile person also wonders, "Why am I not more of a man (or more of a woman)?" The question sometimes asserts itself in the middle of the night as you lie awake saddened by your childlessness. It is important to confront that question by bringing it up in the daytime with your spouse or a counselor.

"What does it mean to you to be a man?" Orlandino often asks her clients. "Does being a man only mean being a father? You're still a man even if your body does not manufacture something."

Female clients are asked the parallel question, "What does it mean to you to be a woman?" Orlandino feels it is important for the infertile woman to explore her notions about sexuality, femininity, and motherhood. "She can then determine what it means to her as an individual to be a woman, rather than what's been dictated to her by society," comments Orlandino.

"People's feelings about their maleness or femaleness are crucial to their understanding of themselves," she adds. "Yet the only time people explore these questions in our society is when something goes wrong and they can't have children."

Ask yourself whether you are being fair to your spouse. Do you listen attentively when he or she is describing feelings? It is not always the healthy spouse who overlooks the needs of the one who is infertile or has a genetic defect. Often it is the spouse with the physical problem who is insensitive to the equally hurting, though physically normal, spouse.

Are you being fair to friends and relatives as well? You may be leaving them at a loss regarding what to do if you send them conflicting signals. Some people say they do not want to be told about a pregnancy or be invited to a baby shower because it upsets them too much, yet they will be upset if excluded.

Much of the emotional trauma can be eased if both of you and your spouse participate in the testing and treatment. Both of you should attend a genetic counseling session. Both should try to go to doctor appointments together. Some women teach their husbands to interpret the temperature chart to detect the most fertile time. That way they do not have to pressure their husbands into a "command performance." Rather, the husband can pick a fertile time that coincides with when he is in the mood. Husbands have also learned to give injections of Pergonal to their wife or administer the artificial insemination of donor semen.

The most important salve to the emotional hurt is good communication and sharing between husband and wife. Some couples find it easier to establish this bond if they attend Resolve sessions or meet with an infertility counselor. Counseling can help in other ways as well. In their study of sixty-two infertile couples who sought counseling, Taymor and Bresnick found a 35 to 65 percent reduction in guilt, anger, and frustration after five or fewer counseling sessions. Long-term therapy (six sessions or more) produced a decrease in these symptoms of 78 to 100 percent.

"Until you have identified and articulated your feelings of anger and loss, you won't be able to make the decision that's most appropriate for you," notes Drew. "Infertility is a shared problem; it is irrelevant which spouse is affected medically. Both have a problem that must be worked on together. If you don't work it out—even if you adopt, have AID, use a surrogate, or have IVF—there's no assurance that the marriage will stay together. There may still be remnants of the guilt and anger."

"You've got to share feelings of blame and the negative feelings as well," agrees Gupta. "If you want to say to your spouse, 'It's your fault I can't have children,' even if it's not physiologically valid, it's better to have it out in the open rather than have the fantasies under the covers.

"It's important and helpful for a couple to let each other know when they're hurting and need comfort and when they need to be left alone," Gupta continues. "People do give clues to how they're feeling—some clam up and some bang around the house. You should teach your husband or wife your clues."

By talking out what bothers you most about your infertility, you can begin to mourn your loss and make decisions about the new direction your life will take. You can ask yourselves whether you really want children or whether you were trying to conceive so that you would not disappoint others.

"Infertility makes people feel that they have lost control," says Orlandino. "But there *are* things they can do. They can remain childless, adopt, have AID, use a surrogate, have *in vitro* fertilization, become a foster parent."

"You can tell you've reached a point where you can make a choice about infertility once you have separated the idea of birthing from the idea of parenting," comments Drew. "Once you realize reproduction doesn't make a parent, then you begin to realize that maybe you do have some choices to get to the goal of parenting."

6 ❧ In Vitro *Fertilization*

When Ellen Casey married in January 1979, she and her husband, Peter, were anxious to start a family. To them, that was really the essence of marriage: sharing your love with the children you bear. After a few months of trying, they got the ominous sense that something was wrong. They did not wait for a year of making love to determine whether they fit the medical definition of infertile but went to a doctor after only a few months.

Ellen underwent a hysterosalpingogram, the X-ray procedure in which dye is injected into the vagina and photographed as it flows through the uterus and fallopian tubes, then out of the tubes into the abdominal cavity. Ellen shivered in her hospital gown, watching the flow of dye through her body on the X-ray monitor. It was taking—in reverse—the same path a baby would take growing inside her and being born.

As Ellen watched, the dye reached an impasse. It got as far as the tubes but no farther. The diagnosis: scarred fallopian tubes, possibly from the IUD Ellen had once used for a few months. She would be unable to conceive because her eggs could not journey down the fallopian tubes for fertilization by Peter's sperm.

Ellen and Peter talked about the results afterward, in hushed tones. The blockage in Ellen's tubes was a roadblock to their having a child. They were barely six months into their marriage and facing what could be the most important decision of their lives. Before they scheduled Ellen for any surgery, they wanted to try to track down the top specialists in the field. They knew that if surgery on the fallopian tubes is to succeed, the first attempt is the critical one. So they started voraciously reading about tubal surgery. In November 1979, they visited a renowned Canadian doctor who performed delicate microsurgery on Ellen's fallopian tubes. The following April she was pregnant, but the pregnancy was ectopic.

They were daunted, but not deterred. They kept reading and learned of the advances being made in laser surgery. In November 1980, Ellen underwent laser surgery in Connecticut. Months went by and no pregnancy.

Where else could they turn, they wondered. Then, on a routine visit, Ellen's local doctor excitedly handed her a copy of a medical journal announcing that Martin Quigley had started an *in vitro* fertilization clinic at the University of Texas Health Science Center in Houston. He made a hopeful suggestion: perhaps the couple would be a good candidate for IVF, *in vitro* fertilization.

With *in vitro* fertilization, a doctor undertakes a laparoscopy to surgically remove an egg from the ovary of a woman. He or she then puts the egg in a petri dish (a small shallow dish with a loose cover) filled with a medium conducive to growth. Next, he or she adds some of the husband's sperm. Once the egg is fertilized, the doctor inserts it without surgery through a tube that passes through the woman's vagina into the uterus. Once in the uterus, the embryo can implant itself and begin to grow like any other embryo. Such offspring are generally referred to as test-tube babies, but as a test tube is never involved, it would actually be more accurate to call them petri-dish progeny.

Although the first IVF baby was not born until 1978, scientific interest in fertilization outside the body dates back decades. A 1937 editorial in the *New England Journal of Medicine* entitled "Conception in a Watch Glass" first suggested fertilizing an egg of a woman outside her body and replacing it in her uterus as a means to alleviate a couple's infertility.

In 1947, scientist M. C. Chang fertilized rabbit ova *in vitro*. Between 1964 and 1972, the same feat was accomplished with eggs from hamsters, mice, cats, rats, guinea pigs, and gerbils. During that time, British scientist Robert Edwards pondered the possibility of fertilizing a human egg outside a woman's body. He made his first attempt in 1965. It was unsuccessful. Years of experimentation followed as he varied different aspects of the procedure. He tried giving women certain hormones before their eggs were removed, used a myriad of treatments on the sperm in an attempt to enhance its fertilizing ability, and concocted various types of culture media to provide the correct stage for fertilization. In one experiment, before undertaking the fertilization, he put the sperm in a chamber lined with porous membranes, and inserted it into a woman's body so that the sperm would have the benefit of being exposed to uterine secretions.

In 1968, Edwards began collaborating with obstetrician Patrick Steptoe, an expert on laparoscopy. a surgical procedure in which a doctor makes a half-inch incision in or below the woman's navel and inserts a laparoscope, a telescopelike instrument through which he can examine her ovaries, fallopian tubes, and uterus. Through another small incision, the doctor can insert another instrument to prick the ovary to remove an egg. In 1969, Edwards and Steptoe reported they had removed an egg from a woman through laparoscopy and successfully fertilized it *in vitro,* which literally means "in glass." Other fertilizations followed and in 1972, they revealed their attempts at implantation. In 1975, they accomplished an implantation, but an ectopic pregnancy occurred.

Edwards' and Steptoe's scientific exploits passed painfully slowly. They had little funding for their efforts; the British Medical Research Council had denied them funds because of doubts about the ethics of their work and qualms about the use of laparoscopy in experimentation. The money they had came primarily from generous individuals (predominantly Americans) and a Ford Foundation grant to Edwards to study *in vitro* fertilization to aid in the development of contraceptives. Ironically, it was this grant for research on *preventing* pregnancy that led (after about one hundred attempts at implantation in various women) to the birth on July 25, 1978 of the world's first test-tube baby, Louise Brown.

• *WHEN IS IVF SUGGESTED?*

The usual reason for using *in vitro* fertilization—as in the case of Ellen Casey or Louise's mother, Lesley Brown—is a tubal problem, blocked or absent fallopian tubes. About 40 percent of all infertile women suffer from tubal problems, most commonly as the result of an infection, for example, from a burst appendix, abdominal surgery, an intrauterine device, or a sexually transmitted disease. The infection can scar the tubes so that an egg cannot pass or it can cause adhesions, closing one end or the other. Tubal damage from an ectopic pregnancy or congenital kinking of the tubes may also impede fertilization within a woman's body.

In the United States alone about 490,000 infertile women have such problems and could possibly be helped by *in vitro* fertilization. The process would also be able to provide a child to women who change their minds after undergoing sterilization by tubal cautery, a hard-to-reverse process.

Dozens of American clinics now offer IVF. Before a couple can be admitted to most clinical programs, the woman must have lost both tubes or both tubes must be blocked. If the tubes are blocked, surgery to repair them through laparoscopy or laparotomy must either be impossible or have been attempted and failed. The couple must have no other infertility factors—in particular, the wife must have at least one ovary and ovulate regularly and the husband must have a normal sperm count. The IVF clinics also set a maximum age for the woman in the couple, generally from thirty-five to thirty-nine. Some clinics also make their services available to couples in which a man has a low sperm count, even if the wife's tubes are perfectly normal.

In vitro fertilization to help a male problem is a significant advance. Because medical science has not focused on male infertility until very recently, very few treatments have been developed to help men. Other than surgery for varicoceles and a few specific treatments that help men who have particular rare maladies affecting sperm production, almost no hope can be offered to men with a low sperm count.

Although it takes only one sperm to fertilize an egg, an estimated ten million at least must enter the woman's body so that 10 percent or so will successfully make the trek through the vagina, cervix, and uterus, to the fallopian tubes. Then one in that million will have a shot at fertilizing the waiting egg. With IVF, though, a man does not need a sperm count of ten million or more. Since the sperm is put directly in the vicinity of the egg, his sperm count can be much lower. For the fertilization of the egg that produced Louise Brown, fewer than a million sperm were used.

At first, doctors were reluctant to offer IVF for couples in which infertility is caused by low sperm counts since they were worried about their scientific credibility. When a woman has serious tubal problems, it is clear that any pregnancy is the result of the IVF process. She could not have gotten pregnant any other way. But when a man has a low sperm count—even dramatically low—there is always a very slight chance that he could have gotten his wife pregnant the natural way. So doctors using IVF for low sperm count run the risk of being told by their scientific colleagues that they did not really cause their claimed IVF pregnancy, nature did.

Dr. Alex Lopata, a successful Australian IVF scientist, already has achieved pregnancies through IVF for couples in which the man has a low sperm count. He also has used IVF for women with endometriosis and couples with immunological incompatibilities or unexplained infertility of over two years' duration. I asked him, "Aren't you worried that your scientific colleagues will say you didn't really cause the birth?"

"Yes, there will be doubters," he replied, "but, for me, it's worth it each time I look into the happy eyes of a couple who have tried so long to have a baby—and now, through this process, have actually succeeded."

• *WHERE TO GO FOR IVF*

Most large medical centers are either currently offering *in vitro* fertilization or are contemplating offering it. Your chances of finding a clinic that will perform IVF on you are ever increasing. Test-tube baby clinics are also flourishing in other countries. There are at least two in England and five in Australia, with others in Italy, France, Sweden, and Germany. At a meeting in Kiel, West Germany, doctors from around the world—Singapore to Sydney—expressed their desire to set up their own clinics. If you can afford the high travel expenses, you might want to apply to one of these programs. Edwards and Steptoe now run a clinic at Bourn Hall, a country manor in Cambridgeshire, England. Among their recent successes: a baby sister for Louise Brown. And on October 21, 1981, an American woman in the program, Laurie Steel, gave birth to a daughter, Samantha, ending her twelve-year quest to become a parent.

Not all foreign clinics welcome Americans, though. The IVF clinic at the Royal Woman's Hospital in Melbourne, Australia, run by Alex Lopata, originally opened its doors to couples from all over the world. Because the Australian government insists on priority for Australian citizens, there is little chance for outsiders who want to be treated at Lopata's clinic.

The number of American clinics is growing rapidly. IVF work is viewed as glamorous and innovative by doctors and scientists. At a recent meeting of the American Fertility Society, it seemed as if every sixth doctor I met (of the hundreds there) wanted to open an IVF clinic. A Norfolk seminar in September 1982 attracted two hundred researchers, representing one hundred different institutions, who planned to offer IVF shortly.

Although any doctor who wanted to could attempt *in vitro* fertilization, it takes a special combination of expertise and talent to make the process actually work. The average gynecologist or obstetrician—or even the better-than-average infertility specialist—may try to provide IVF but probably will not succeed. To save yourself the time, trouble, pain, and disappointment of IVF performed by less than the very best hands, it is important to choose your program well. When you contact a program, ask about the number and type of people they have on staff (a team approach of an endocrinologist, gynecologist, obstetrician, biologist, and lab technicians is best). Ask how long they have been offering IVF, how many couples they have treated, and how many successes they have had so far. Then you can make a better informed decision about whether to join a particular program.

Also make sure the doctor you choose does not feel it necessary to sterilize you by closing up your tubes before you undergo IVF. Some doctors actually advocate that approach, partly because they do not wish their patients to have to suffer through an ectopic pregnancy. But a selfish motivation is present, too; if your tubes are surgically closed you will not be able to conceive naturally. Therefore the doctor can take full credit for any subsequent pregnancy.

Dr. Ian Craft, an *in vitro* specialist in England, argues against pre-IVF sterilizations. He believes an ectopic pregnancy after IVF is unlikely if the embryo is transferred in a small amount of fluid and is not placed close to the tube when it is implanted. He also maintains that infertile patients should not be subjected to the additional stress of sterilization. "It would be difficult to justify its performance for women having in vitro fertilisation for unexplained infertility in whom the fallopian tubes are normal," wrote Craft with colleagues Fraser McLeod and Keith Edmonds in the British medical journal *Lancet.* "A situation could occur whereby attempted in vitro fertilisation might be unsuccessful and yet pregnancy might occur naturally in a subsequent untreated cycle."

Most American programs estimate that the couple's medical costs will be about $4,000 to $5,000 per attempt at *in vitro* fertilization. Some programs require the couple to agree to make at least four attempts, making entry into a program very expensive. Except for some initial diagnostic procedures, the costs are not usually covered by insurance. An editorial in an influential insurance magazine may change that, however. The editorial in *Business Insurance* called for insurance companies to cover the costs an infertile couple incurs in conceiving a child with laboratory aid. The editorial criticized insurers for their seeming insensitivity in labeling IVF not necessary: "Try telling a childless couple that laboratory fertilization, which may be the only way they can have a family, is non-necessary. Without insurance, the cost of the procedure . . . might prevent a couple from proceeding."

In addition to the medical costs, you will incur extensive travel costs if you go to a clinic that is out of state or out of the country. If you undergo IVF at the Norfolk clinic, you and your husband will have to travel there for an initial visit and diagnostic tests, return each time an egg is removed and fertilization and implantation is attempted, and perhaps again for the delivery of the baby. (On the last visit the wife could go alone, but what husband would want to miss out on the excitement of seeing his seconds-old child and getting the chance to pass out cigars?)

• *WHAT THE IVF PROGRAM ENTAILS*

The process of IVF is so new that every clinic has a slightly different way of performing it. All programs have five general phases, though: diagnosis, recovery of an egg, fertilization, implantation, and obstetrical care.

In most programs, a diagnostic laparoscopy is required, even if the woman has already undergone the procedure elsewhere. This is done under general anesthesia in a hospital operating room. The doctor makes a small incision near the navel and inserts a long, thin telescopelike instrument into the woman's abdomen so that he can look at the woman's ovaries and, if she has any, her tubes. This is the critical juncture at which the doctor will decide whether the woman actually is a good candidate for IVF. The crucial question is whether her ovaries are accessible so that the doctor will easily be able to draw an egg out. In some cases the task is just too difficult—the ovaries are covered with adhesions, or are attached to some other body organ so that the doctor would not be able to remove the egg for *in vitro* fertilization. Ellen Casey was lucky; her diagnostic laparoscopy showed that one ovary was 80 percent accessible and the other 60 percent accessible, making her a good candidate for IVF.

Although most doctors do not schedule the diagnostic laparoscopy for any particular time in the cycle, some doctors are anxious not to let any opportunity go by for helping a couple get pregnant. They schedule the procedure for a time slightly before the woman is due to ovulate. On the morning of the procedure, the woman and her husband are told to make love so that some of his sperm would be in her uterus or the lower part of her fallopian tubes at the time of the surgery. That way, if the doctor happened to be doing the laparoscopy at the precise time of the month when an egg was ready to burst forth from the patient's ovaries, he or she would transfer that egg from the ovary to the lower part of the fallopian tube or the uterus, where it might become fertilized *in vivo* ("in the living body").

LOOKING FOR AN EGG

For the 80 percent of the IVF couples who are not eliminated from an IVF program by the diagnostic laparoscopy, the true wonders of modern science are revealed in the next few steps of the process. The key is to remove an egg from the woman's body at a critical point: when it is mature enough so that it will be fertilized but not so mature that it has already left its nurturing nest in the ovary. "According to certain research, there is only a three- to four-hour time span each month when the egg is in precisely the right stage for removal," explains Martin Quigley.

When doctors first started doing *in vitro* fertilization they would wait patiently through the woman's natural cycle until she produced an egg. Now doctors give women fertility drugs so they can more accurately time the egg recovery and so that multiple eggs will be produced, increasing the chances of fertilization and subsequent pregnancy.

When pioneering IVF researchers Steptoe and Edwards started collaborating, the timing problem of getting an egg at the precise moment it was ready was heightened by the fact that they lived and worked 180 miles apart. Steptoe had an obstetrical position at a small country hospital in the old textile mill town of Oldham in the northwest region of England. Edwards taught physiology at Cambridge University. When the urine tests of a patient at the Oldham Hospital showed she would be ovulating within the next half day, Steptoe would call Edwards, day or night, and Edwards would hop into a car and drive the bumpy back roads to take his place at Steptoe's side. They had fixed up a small supply room next to the hospital operating room as a laboratory. When Steptoe removed the fluid from a woman's ovaries, Edwards could immediately examine it and put any egg into a dish with a special culture to nourish it to begin readying it for fertilization.

As they collaborated for a number of years, the two refined their procedure. They installed an intercom system between the laboratory and the operating room so that Edwards could immediately let Steptoe know if there was an egg in the fluid he had withdrawn. They got so adept at the procedure that, by the time Lesley Brown became their patient, the time that elapsed from Steptoe's locating a ripening follicle to Edwards' placement of the egg in culture was a mere two minutes.

The difficulty of tracing a woman's cycle and pinpointing exactly when ovulation will occur has led IVF doctors to induce ovulation with hormones. Among other benefits, this means the full team of IVF staff need not be on call twenty-four hours a day, as they must be when the egg is recovered during a woman's natural cycle.

The various IVF programs differ in the hormones they use to stimulate ovulation. Some use Pergonal, others use a milder drug, clomiphene citrate, still others use a combination of the two. Doctors Howard and Georgeanna Jones at the Norfolk clinic give their patients Pergonal to control ovulation. Also, the women are injected with HCG thirty-six hours before laparoscopy is expected to take place. Pergonal has the effect of ripening several eggs and increases the chance that at least one egg will be successfully recovered and fertilized. In the case of Judy Carr, America's first test-tube baby mother, Pergonal led to the production of two eggs—one not fully developed but the other perfect.

In Quigley's program in Houston, the woman is given clomiphene citrate on days five to nine of her cycle. As in the Norfolk program, HCG is given thirty-six hours before the scheduled laparoscopy. Quigley teaches the husband to give the wife the shot, instructing him to do it around midnight. This had led to some nervous but humorous scenes across the bedrooms of Texas. "One night I was awakened by a call from a sheepish husband," recalls Quigley. "He told me that he tried to give the shot but missed entirely and squirted the drug across the room."

To help pinpoint the expected time of ovulation, Quigley uses an ultrasound test, a painless procedure in which sound waves are bounced off a woman's abdomen, resulting in a computerized picture of her ovaries on a screen. By assessing the size and shape of the ovarian follicles, Quigley can determine the best time to attempt to collect the eggs. He tries to snare them through laparoscopy shortly before they would otherwise burst from the ovaries.

Once it appears that the woman will ovulate in a few hours, she is admitted to the hospital for the laparoscopy to remove all the ripe eggs. Shortly before her laparoscopy, one of Quigley's patients surprised him with an unusual gift. She handed him an egg carton. She had crossed out the name of the farm and written in the doctor's so the carton now read "Quigley's Eggs."

"Please fill this up for me," she requested.

EGG RETRIEVAL

For the egg retrieval process, the woman is given a general anesthesia and wheeled into an operating room for a laparoscopy. Through the laparoscope, the doctor views the ovaries, seeking the characteristic little bump that indicates an egg has matured in its follicle and is ready to leave the ovaries. Through another incision, the doctor inserts a hollow needlelike instrument to prick each bump and withdraw the fluid it contains. In some IVF programs, a third incision is made to insert another needlelike instrument that gently pushes aside the fallopian tubes or any other organ that gets in the way of access to the ovaries. The incisions are small and the doctor can go into those incisions made during the diagnostic laparoscopy, so that the woman will have no more than three tiny scars.

In the IVF program at Mt. Sinai Hospital in Chicago, an alternative to laparoscopy known as vaginal egg retrieval has been used in a few instances to collect the eggs. The vaginal wall is numbed with a local anesthetic and then a needle is inserted into the vagina and through the vaginal wall to puncture the ovary and retrieve an egg. The doctor checks an ultrasound image of the woman's pelvic cavity so that he can aim for a ripe follicle.

Vaginal egg retrieval was developed to extend IVF to women whose ovaries were not accessible through traditional laparoscopy, but Dr. Norbert Gleicher, chairman of obstetrics at Mt. Sinai Hospital, feels it could replace laparoscopic egg retrieval. He feels that the procedure has fewer risks and could be less costly than surgical removal of the eggs. One drawback is that vaginal egg retrieval seems to permit fewer eggs to be removed per cycle—about two compared to the average of five removed through a laparoscopy procedure.

Dr. Jan Friberg, Director of the Division of Reproductive Endocrinology/Infertility at Mt. Sinai, describes another alternative to laparoscopy that they are currently exploring—transcutaneous needle aspiration. Ultrasound is used to locate the ripening follicle and then a long needle is inserted directly into the women's abdomen into the follicle to withdraw the egg. "The successful application of this procedure could mean that *in vitro* fertilization could move out of the hospitals into private practice," says Friberg.

Since the eggs removed through laparoscopy or vaginal egg retrieval are so small that they are invisible to the naked eye, the doctor cannot be sure that he or she has actually gotten any eggs until the fluid has been examined under a microscope. In the Houston program, the laboratory is located very close to the operating room. While Ellen Casey was undergoing laparoscopy, her husband, Peter, waited anxiously in the lab. Each time Quigley withdrew fluid from one of Ellen's ripe ovarian follicles, a technician would rush it to the lab and examine it under the microscope. On a closed circuit television, Peter could see exactly what the technician could see. He watched with excitement each time the technician scanned a new batch of fluid. He felt their chances of a pregnancy were good. Quigley had recovered five of Ellen's eggs.

After a short period of time in the recovery room, Ellen felt well enough to leave the hospital. The laparoscopy is a safe enough procedure that hospitalization that evening is not required. Peter and Ellen went back to their hotel to celebrate—and await the news about whether any of the eggs had been fertilized.

FERTILIZATION

About two hours before the woman is scheduled to undergo the laparoscopy (or in some programs, a few hours after the surgery), her husband is asked to do his part. He is given a small plastic specimen cup, pointed to a bathroom, and asked to produce some semen.

In the laboratory the schedule for the egg and sperm is much the same as it would be in the woman's body. The egg continues to develop for about five hours in a solution of salts, amino acids, vitamins, and human blood serum, so that it fully matures and is able to be fertilized.

The sperm is washed in the same culture medium used for the egg. Then each egg is introduced to about 20,000 to 500,000 sperm in a shallow plastic dish. Each dish is put into an incubator set at body heat.

If you were to view the fertilization process through the microscope, you would be truly amazed. While the egg sits regally and firmly, the area around it is abuzz with activity. Sperm stream up to it from all directions, moving their tails repeatedly. Some move toward the egg head on, others seem to be chasing their tails in circles, Finally, one breaks the surface of the egg like a graceful swimmer entering a calm pond. The head of the sperm disappears under the surface of the egg, the tail smoothly following. Through a process not yet fully understood, this union of egg and sperm (whether in the body or outside of it) appears to set off a particular chemical reaction so that no other sperm can enter the egg.

The fertilized egg, the first cell of that new human being, next divides, creating two cells. They each divide again, achieving four. This is the stage at which many IVF doctors transfer the fertilized embryo into the mother's body. In the case of Judy Carr, a four-cell embryo was implanted on her twenty-eighth birthday, but the real present did not come until nine months later, when that embryo had grown and entered the world as the newborn Elizabeth.

IMPLANTATION

The implantation itself is a technically simple procedure. Anesthesia is not required and the whole process takes only a few minutes. The woman assumes a position similar to that of a routine pelvic examination, and a thin rubber tube containing fluid and the fertilized egg is inserted into her vagina and up through her cervix. Its contents are gently expelled into her uterus. If more than one of her eggs has successfully been fertilized, they are all implanted at the same time. In Australia, Canada, and the United States this has led to the birth of test-tube twins. An Australian woman in June 1983 gave birth to the world's first set of test-tube triplets.

Ellen Casey's implantation took place before noon, but Steptoe and Edwards prefer to do their implantations in the evening. Maybe it's a matter of superstition, since, in their early research, the two implantations that had been done at night led to pregnancies, while implantations done at other times did not. Perhaps science plays a part as well, though, since Edwards points out that in the evening the hormones necessary for sustaining a pregnancy are at their highest level. The adrenal glands, controlling the body's day-to-day activity, are least active, slowing down the body's processes and creating a more restful home for the embryo.

At the Bourn Hall clinic run by Steptoe and Edwards, the night implantation has become somewhat of a romantic ritual, with the woman dressing up for the occasion. When it was Laurie Steel's turn, she carefully combed her long blonde hair, put on makeup, and slipped into a magenta velvet gown. In Quigley's clinic in Houston, the husband usually joins the wife in the room for the implantation, so the couple can experience the special time together. Peter and Ellen Casey quietly held hands during the implantation.

Even without these romantic trappings, the women involved in *in vitro* fertilization feel something special about the moment the fertilized egg enters their womb. "That was a wonderful experience," exclaimed Lesley Brown as soon as the implantation took place.

AFTER IMPLANTATION

Once the embryo is inside its mother, the normal bodily processes take over to nurture it. The woman is usually advised to remain in bed for the first twenty-four hours. "I was afraid to even move," recalls Ellen Casey. "After twenty-four hours, when they told me I could go, I did not want to get out of the bed. I had the unrealistic fear the embryo might fall to the floor."

For the first week or so of an IVF pregnancy, doctors watch the process closely. The hormone primarily responsible for the safety and comfort of the early embryo is progesterone, which is produced by the corpus luteum in the follicle from which the egg has emerged. There is some risk that puncturing the follicle to remove an egg by laparoscopy will hamper it so that it will not meet all the hormonal needs of the developing embryo. The doctor therefore may order frequent blood tests beginning three days after implantation and prescribe injections or vaginal suppositories of progesterone if it appears that the follicle is not producing enough.

AMNIOCENTESIS AND DELIVERY

As their IVF pregnancy continues, some couples begin to wonder about the health of their developing child. This, of course, is a normal concern for all parents-to-be, but IVF couples sometimes have an added fear—what if the IVF process itself caused the child to be deformed or unhealthy?

Luckily, nature thoughtfully provided added protection to the preimplantation embryo. Research with animals found that there is very little risk of an abnormality caused by the *in vitro* fertilization process. Experimenters exposed animal embryos to heat, freezing temperatures, radiation, toxins, viruses, and other harsh processes and contaminants. The *in vitro* embryos were highly resistant to these assaults; there was no increase in abnormalities. Although extensive studies have not been performed with humans, initial research has found that the human egg is one of the most resistant.

Of course, even if the embryo were developing with a gross defect, a woman's body is fairly good at screening out abnormal embryos. (In fact, 99.3 percent to 99.5 percent of chromosomally abnormal fetuses created through regular intercourse perish or are spontaneously aborted during pregnancy.) Nevertheless, with their initial IVF pregnancies, Steptoe and Edwards felt it necessary to ask the women to undergo amniocentesis in their fourth month so that the fluid could be analyzed to see if the fetus was free of certain genetic defects.

Amniocentesis is not without risk. As many as one in a thousand to one in a hundred fetuses will be harmed by the process. One Australian IVF patient miscarried shortly after amniocentesis, causing doctors there to rethink their position on the procedure.

Now the test is generally no longer done routinely, either in Australia or the United States. Ellen Casey did not undergo amniocentesis, although she could have if she had been especially worried about her baby's genetic makeup.

The prime malady screened for through amniocentesis is Down's syndrome, which becomes increasingly common as the mother's age increases. At age thirty, a woman has a one in eight hundred chance of giving birth to a child with Down's syndrome; by age thirty-five the risk rises to one in three hundred. At age forty, it is one in one hundred. Since the women undergoing IVF are generally under age thirty-five, the need for amniocentesis is less pressing, as they are at a lesser risk of having an affected child than are older women. Of the IVF children born to date, most have been healthy except for two born with heart defects that required surgery soon after birth. So far there is absolutely no evidence that IVF children have a greater risk of abnormality than children conceived naturally.

Like all infertile women who subsequently become pregnant, IVF mothers feel that they are carrying a fragile jewel within them. In the case of IVF, though, the doctors may share that feeling. Test-tube babies are still so rare that the doctors are extra cautious in handling their delivery. Howard Jones, for example, delivered Elizabeth Carr by a Caesarean section to ease her transition into the world as much as possible. But Alex Lopata at his Australian clinic does not like to interfere with the initial bonding of the mother and child. His IVF patients give birth naturally.

• *THE EMOTIONAL ASPECTS OF IVF*

For many couples, IVF brings with it an emotional rainbow, with feelings of different intensities overlapping one another. With the announcement of Louise Brown's birth, hundreds of thousands of couples around the world felt an unparalled hope in place of that empty ache of childlessness. Before you dash off that letter to the nearest IVF clinic or one of the other ones, do your best to make sure you are not engaging in false hope. See a specialist to make sure that IVF is the answer to your problem. "The most heartbreaking thing that we're finding" says Quigley of himself and the other test-tube baby doctors, "is the woman who is mistakenly on a waiting list for an IVF for months and months because her problem was not adequately diagnosed by the referring doctor." The wait, the extra period of stress, the possible breakup in the marriage all could have been avoided by an accurate initial diagnosis. Moreover, when the test-tube baby doctors are wasting time on a workup on someone who could have been helped, with a higher success rate, by traditional means, a deserving couple for whom IVF is the only hope is forced to wait.

Once you enter an IVF program, it is as if you were watching a high-powered medical research show. Never before have so many medical professionals of such talent joined together to help a couple produce a child. Electricity is in the air as you enter the clinic and talk to the receptionists, nurses, doctors, and scientists in the program; they are thrilled by their work in this brave new field. For every couple in the world, having their baby is a special, miraculous, one-of-a-kind experience. Usually their obstetrician, who has delivered hundreds of babies or more, is calm about the process. In an IVF program, you will find the doctors as excited as you are—maybe even more so. When Quigley waits for a pregnancy test of one of his IVF patients, he is as anxious as any hopeful father-to-be.

"Normally, a pregnancy is achieved by just you and your husband," comments Ellen Casey. "But *in vitro* fertilization takes it out of the personal realm and puts it into the medical realm. This could make it feel mechanical, but I never had that feeling at all. The members of the Houston clinic really love you and care for you."

Part of the reason Ellen feels so positive about the IVF process is that every stage in the procedure had been carefully explained to her. She had been given a tour of the room where her egg would be fertilized. And since her husband was involved in every step, the conception of the child was a mutual, loving act. "I've never been through anything like that before," enthuses Peter Casey. "It was wonderful. Everyone in the process was so close and supportive. It was like going down to be with family."

IN VITRO FERTILIZATION • 137

At first, Peter was cautious. "Ellen had gone through pure hell trying to have a baby, with microsurgery, laser surgery, and everything else," Peter recounts. "The odds were astronomically against us and I didn't want to see her disappointed again."

At a world conference on IVF in 1980, biologist E.S.E. Hafez of Wayne State University reported that IVF had been attempted on twenty thousand women at that point, but there had been only three proven births—or a success rate of .015 percent.

In the past few years, refinement of the IVF techniques has improved the success rate markedly. Reports in medical journals and at meetings of the American Fertility Society indicate that pregnancies occur 10 to 20 percent of the time—one or two chances in ten.

The IVF practitioners counsel couples that the reproductive process is a complicated one and, just as in natural conception, the IVF conception may encounter difficulties at any of a number of stages. The time of ovulation may be misjudged or may be unpredictable or ovulation may not occur in the monitored cycle, thus precluding any attempt at obtaining an egg. Cleavage or cell division of the fertilized egg may not occur. The embryo may not develop normally. Implantation may not occur. If pregnancy is successfully established, miscarriage, ectopic pregnancy, stillbirth, or birth defects may occur (even though there is no indication that the occurrence of these is increased by the procedure). Extensive research in the test-tube baby centers across the country, including tests involving animals, aims at minimizing these potential roadblocks to an IVF pregnancy.

Even if *in vitro* fertilization develops to the point where it is as efficient and successful as fertilization in the body, you will not be guaranteed a child every time you have an egg removed. According to research on fertilization occurring within the body, there is only a 32 percent chance that a baby will result when egg meets sperm. Of one hundred instances when that occurs, in sixteen the egg will fail to fertilize, in fifteen a fertilized egg will fail to implant, in twenty-seven the embryo will abort before the woman even notices she is pregnant, and in an additional ten, spontaneous abortion (miscarriage) will occur later.

So do not despair if the IVF process does not work for you the first month you try it. Once you are in an IVF program, the doctors will keep trying, sometimes as soon as the following month if you wish. Although the Houston clinic has a maximum of three tries per couple (imposed by the University of Texas Health Science Center's Committee for the Protection of Human Subjects, which must vote on all research at the institution), other clinics will apparently keep trying indefinitely. One Norfolk patient has already undergone IVF five times.

For the couples who do achieve a pregnancy through IVF, the thrill is extraordinary. In addition, there are no mixed feelings as sometimes occur in the other reproductive technologies, where there is fear that the sperm donor or egg donor or surrogate will somehow make a claim on your child. The IVF doctors and scientists have no basis to sue you to get it back. So when the baby is born, the couples' reaction to the professionals is one of immense gratitude. "Dr. Quigley is like another parent to our baby," acknowledges Ellen Casey. "We feel a debt of gratitude and love toward him that we will never ever experience in any other way in our life."

• *SOCIETY'S REACTION TO IVF*

In their joy at potential parenthood—and in the excitement they share with their families and the clinic staff—IVF couples are sometimes unprepared for the controversy and notoriety that surrounds the process. Unlike artificial insemination, which was introduced as an infertility practice with utmost secrecy, *in vitro* fertilization came into the world with widespread publicity. Newspapers, magazines, and television stations treated the impending birth of a baby to John and Lesley Brown as an extraordinary event. When the pregnant Mrs. Brown was hospitalized, press people dressed up as boiler makers, plumbers, and window cleaners to sneak into the hospital to try to interview or photograph her. One exasperated hospital representative complained: "It seems as if you move anything, there is a reporter behind it." The newspapers even surreptitiously obtained—and printed—reports of confidential medical tests that had been performed on Lesley to monitor the development of the child within her. One day the shock of reading a newspaper report drastically raised Lesley's blood pressure. "Is it true that my baby nearly died yesterday?" she asked Patrick Steptoe, in tears. "Is it true? Will it happen again?"

Steptoe assured her all was well and, true to his word, delivered the healthy baby Louise a few weeks later. The media stepped up its coverage, breathlessly reporting the birth of Louise Brown with the detail usually reserved for a major political event, a journey in space, or the marriage of royalty. Newspapers in every language reported Louise Brown's worldly debut. Or was it really an encore? She had been in the world before, when she was eight cells old, no bigger than the dot at the end of this sentence.

A month after Louise's birth, in August 1978, *Parents* magazine sponsored a Harris poll of around fifteen hundred American women. Eighty-five percent of the women said they felt IVF should be an option for infertile women. Overall, 58 percent of the women said they would themselves consider using IVF. Among younger women, age eighteen to thirty-nine, the number was even higher (61 percent). Most of the women in the poll still viewed the procedure somewhat tentatively, saying that given a choice, they would pick adoption (57 percent) over IVF (21 percent).

A similar Gallup poll of both men and women, also taken in August 1978, found that 60 percent favored the availability of the procedure to anyone who needed and wanted it. Gallup found that "an extraordinary 93 percent had heard or read about the baby." Forty-two percent could fully and correctly explain *in vitro* fertilization. Despite the apparent support of IVF, some people misunderstand the process. "When people found out I was several months pregnant after having *in vitro* fertilization, they said things like 'Who's the father?' or 'Where's the baby?' thinking it was growing in some jar somewhere like in 1984," Ellen Casey reports.

There are also a number of vocal opponents to the *in vitro* fertilization procedure. Paul Ramsey, a professor of religion at

Princeton, declared he half-hoped the first test-tube baby would be deformed and put up for public display, apparently to discourage others from undertaking the process.

When Howard and Georgeanna Jones proposed to open an IVF clinic in Norfolk, Virginia, the Tidewater chapter of the Virginia Society for Human Life tried several tactics to prevent it. The Tidewater antiabortion group first took their case to the state health commissioner in an attempt to prevent the Joneses from receiving approval to open the clinic. Once the clinic was established, the antiabortion group mailed hundreds of petitions urging that tax money be withdrawn from the Eastern Virginia Medical School until it severed its tie with the Joneses' test-tube baby clinic.

One of the commonly voiced oppositions to IVF is that it is destructive of the family. There is the concern that IVF turns procreation from a loving, personal experience into a laboratory process. But the couples using IVF are not deliberately foregoing natural conception; they have no other choice.

"*In vitro* fertilization is the most profamily thing I can think of," maintains Ellen Casey. "No one has tried harder to get a baby than someone in an *in vitro* program. There has been so much pain and heartache and searching for someone who has turned to *in vitro* fertilization. There's no more wanted baby in the world than an *in vitro* baby."

Opponents of IVF also suggest that it is like playing God. "If God did not want it to happen, it would never work," responds Casey. "It's a blessing from God. It's made me far more religious than I have ever been before."

Because IVF is for certain couples the only means of having their own children, it seems strange that the right-to-life people oppose it. As Clifford Grobstein, professor of biological science and public policy at the University of California at San Diego, points out, IVF is not destructive of the family. "On the contrary," he writes in his book *From Chance to Purpose: An Appraisal of External Human Fertilization,* "the immediate purpose is to create a family, an objective exactly opposite to the concern expressed."

Infertile couples who stand to benefit from IVF are stunned at the charge that it is antifamily. As Roger Carr, the father of the first test-tube baby born in America, told a PBS reporter, "I just can't possibly understand how anyone could think that what the Joneses have done, or what was done in England . . . I don't see how anybody could say that this is immoral, or that people are playing God. I mean, to me, if they take our little baby when it's born and they hold it in their hands how can anybody say that that is wrong?"

Howard Jones, who along with his wife, Georgeanna Jones, founded the Norfolk clinic, takes issue with the assertion that IVF is unethical because science does not have the right to manipulate nature. "Actually, every request of a physician to diagnose and treat disease is a request to manipulate nature," asserts Jones. "If it is ethically acceptable to seek medical care for a reproductive disorder, it is ethically acceptable to seek care which requires *in vitro* fertilization."

Lord Kilbrandon, a British attorney, noted that IVF "is analogous to a Caesarean birth: simply an artificial means of organizing an ordinary birth." Dr. John Marlow, of Columbia Hospital for Women in Washington, D.C., points out that premature babies are maintained in an artificial environment, an incubator, for up to twenty weeks, much longer than the two to six days an IVF embryo is in its artificial environment, the petri dish.

Edwards and Steptoe also cringe at the notion that what they are doing is unethical: "We believe that our studies conform with the Hippocratic oath in that they are for the benefit of patient and not for their hurt or for any wrong—indeed we believe they hold out the prospect of widespread benefit."

Some IVF participants have made themselves available to the media or formed special IVF patients groups to combat the impression that the process is somehow unseemly. Before Dr. Alan DeCherney established his *in vitro* fertilization clinic at the Yale School of Medicine, he traveled throughout Connecticut, speaking at churches and civic groups to explain exactly what he planned to do so that there would be no misconceptions. His fine medical school training had not prepared him for the selling job he would have to do to convince the people of Connecticut that what he was doing was not morally wrong. "I even had to debate a nun on television," recalls DeCherney. "I was terrified about doing it."

The pressures on researchers are enormous. Steptoe and Edwards were distraught when, after they published reports of their early attempts to fertilize eggs outside a woman's body, the Archbishop of Liverpool denounced their work as "morally wrong."

Alex Lopata, a kind and gentle man, heads a successful Australian IVF clinic. Imagine his dismay when he learned that priests were actually staging a hunger strike in his hospital lobby to protest his work! Lopata's patients had to walk past this human barrier whenever they wanted to see him. The strain in his lab and clinic was tremendous. Finally, a slight young woman, one of Lopata's IVF patients, calmly walked into the heat of the protest. She looked a priest directly in the eye and asked quietly, "Why don't you want me to have this baby?"

To be fair, the issue for many opponents of IVF is not wanting to stop the birth of a *particular* baby or dash the dreams of an infertile couple. Rather, they are concerned about the changes in society that they think *in vitro* fertilization will lead to. Among their concerns: fears that acceptance of IVF will lead to diminished respect for human life and various attempts to engineer a better race.

Biologist and ethicist Leon Kass hypothesizes about the dehumanizing effect IVF will have on the researchers. Kass urges that we should "be concerned about the effects on the attitude toward and respect for human life engendered in persons who are engaged in such research."

Contrary to Kass' fears, doctors and scientists performing IVF to bring children to infertile couples have not become dehumanized. To them, as much as to the layperson, the fertilization taking place under the microscope is a miracle. The staff of the infertility clinics treat the embryo with the respect that they would any "patient" as they struggle valiantly to give that embryo every chance to come into the world.

In research, the issues are slightly different. Some scientists want to use fertilized eggs, not to bring a child into the home of a previously infertile couple, but to study them to learn more about the reproductive process so that they can improve treatment of infertile couples or design better contraceptives. Other scientists would like to use fertilized human eggs that will not be re-implanted to test new drugs or chemicals for toxicity. In this way, they say, a tragedy like the thalidomide disaster might be averted.

Will experimenting on embryos— and then discarding them— cause scientists to lose respect for human life in general? Much depends on the scientists' personal, moral, and religious convictions. For researcher Dr. R. F. Harrison of Dublin, Ireland, IVF is fraught with questions because he views the embryo as a human being. "Surely there is no problem with embryo transfer when it actually works," explains Harrison. "But what worries me is, if I am experimenting, trying embryo transfer, and I get to the six- to eight-cell stage and then I deliberately stop that, I'm killing a human life."

Other researchers and ethicists express an equally heartfelt contrary conclusion. They believe that it shows no disrespect to do research with a fertilized egg, even after it has begun dividing, since they do not view that cluster of cells as a person. Samuel Gorovitz, for example, asserts: "The status of the embryo is not equivalent to that of a person, a child, an infant, or a fetus. . . ." Gorovitz, a philosophy professor at the University of Maryland, believes that protectable personhood does not begin until the fetus develops the capacity to respond to sensory stimuli, between the eighth and tenth week of gestation.

Kass' argument that IVF will necessarily lead to a devaluation of respect for other lives (such as the elderly or newborns with genetic defects) is the same argument that was made against the widespread availability of abortion. A decade after the U.S. Supreme Court decision sanctioning abortion, however, society's respect for the vulnerable is still intact.

Kass also worries about other potential applications of the IVF procedure. He fears that IVF will lead to procreation by design, with parents picking the traits they want in their offspring. Kass predicts that IVF will give rise to ova and embryos being "banked" and sold for commercial purposes. Such a development is scientifically possible. In fact, E.S.E. Hafez predicts that it will be possible to have an embryo supermarket. According to Hafez, the purchaser would be able to select an embryo knowing in advance the "color of the baby's eyes and hair, its sex, its probable size at maturity, and its probable I.Q."

Critics of IVF also suggest that once scientists begin isolating an egg and sperm in a laboratory, they may try crossing species—for example, using an ape embryo and human sperm or vice versa. Nobel Prize winner J.B.S. Haldane suggested altering certain men (through gene grafts on the embryo) so that they had monkey traits, including long arms and a stooped posture. These hybrids could then serve as astronauts. Wrote Haldane: "A gibbon is better adapted than a man for life in a low gravitational field such as that of a spaceship, an asteroid, or perhaps even the moon. Gene grafting may make it possible to incorporate such features into human stock."

In a less complex experiment, in the late 1960s, Chinese surgeon Ji Yongxiang successfully fertilized a chimpanzee with human sperm to create a "near human ape" to perform simple tasks. The pregnancy was terminated when rioters destroyed his lab, but Yongxiang, who believes that the world is ready for animal-human hybrids, advocates trying again.

Already, a law journal article has raised the questions about whether hybrids will have the same legal rights as humans. If the hybrid is half human will it have the right to vote? What about its offspring, who might be only a quarter human?

Luckily, the day of the superchild or the apeperson is not yet here—and may never come. The couple seeking IVF are not asking for the sperm of an Einstein and the egg of a Madame Curie or certain genetic traits of a cheetah. Rather, they are trying desperately for the chance to have their own biological child, with whatever foibles and flaws, beauty and wit that the magic combination of their own genes creates. Yes, science is moving extraordinarily quickly. As a society, it is important for us to start thinking about the science-fictionlike scenarios that may be just around the corner. There may indeed be some practices we might wish to ban, such as experiments across species. But it seems unfair to infertile couples to ban all use of IVF merely because of fear that it will launch us into a nightmare world.

After all, IVF may not necessarily lead to these practices, and these practices may take hold even if IVF were banned. The Chinese attempt to merge human and ape did not rely on IVF—and even if IVF with its laparoscopy component were banned, scientists could use eggs from the ovaries of women whose ovaries had been removed in the course of a complete hysterectomy. What would the opponents then propose—that hysterectomy (a necessary medical procedure) be banned on the off chance that a scientist may decide to breed a genius hybrid with the egg? For a truly just law it seems wise to recognize and allow the beneficial uses of IVF and guard against those that would thwart individual rights.

• *THE ETHICAL ISSUES OF IVF*

The process of unraveling the intricate ethical issues surrounding IVF has occupied not only scientists and the public but also the federal government. In 1974, Dr. Pierre Soupart, a professor at Vanderbilt University, submitted an application for funding to the National Institutes of Health (NIH). Two years earlier, in 1972, he had been the first American scientist to prove he could fertilize a human egg *in vitro*. In his 1974 funding request, he proposed a three-year, $375,000 study to determine the safety of *in vitro* fertilization. With the cooperation of women who were undergoing gynecological surgery for other reasons and would donate eggs, Soupart planned to fertilize 450 eggs, grow them for around six days, and study their chromosomes to see whether the *in vitro* fertilization process caused any chromosomal abnormality. Soupart's proposal was for research only; he did not intend to implant any fertilized embryos.

In the spring of 1975, Soupart learned that NIH would grant his funding if the Ethics Advisory Board (EAB) of the Department of Health, Education and Welfare determined that the research was ethical. A 1975 federal law had provided for the creation of EAB; however, it took two years for the government to appoint members. Not until 1978 did the board begin its deliberation of

Soupart's proposal. The EAB had before it the task of studying IVF, analyzing all the arguments pro and con, and making suggestions for a government policy on IVF. The Secretary of HEW (at that time, Joseph Califano) did not want the board to limit its consideration to Soupart's proposal. Rather, he wanted the board to undertake a massive fact-finding mission about the scientific, ethical, legal, and social issues raised by IVF.

The fifteen-member board, which included physicians, medical ethicists, three lawyers, a psychiatrist, and three civic leaders, worked from May 1978 to May 1979 gathering information and preparing their report. They held hearings across the nation, taking testimony from medical and scientific experts, theologians, people with infertility problems, concerned individuals, professional organizations, and various special interest groups. They received two thousand pieces of correspondence to guide them in their quest. They hired consultants to prepare reports on the massive literature that existed about IVF. The EAB's task took on an added importance when, two months after they began their analysis of the IVF issues, baby Louise was born in England. (Ironically, if Soupart had been given the funding when he initially asked for it, the first test-tube baby might have been American.)

The board never felt its task was an easy one. Board members compassionately and thoughtfully weighed the facts and worked their way to a number of conclusions. They recognized the possibility for abuse with this technology as there is, they pointed out, with any technology. The board concluded, however, that "a broad prohibition of research involving human *in vitro* fertilization is neither justified nor wise."

The EAB also reported that "concerns regarding the moral status of the embryo and the potential long-range consequences of this research were among the most difficult that confronted the Board." After painstakingly careful thought, though, the board decided that research involving human *in vitro* fertilization was both acceptable from an ethical viewpoint and worthy of federal support. "After much analysis and discussion regarding both scientific data and the moral status of the embryo," the EAB concluded "that the human embryo is entitled to profound respect; but this respect does not necessarily encompass the full legal and moral rights attributed to persons."

The board also concluded that conduct of research involving human IVF designed to establish the safety and effectiveness of the procedures should be subject to certain restrictions. One condition is that the embryo would be sustained no longer than fourteen days after fertilization. Another is that the public be advised if "evidence begins to show that the procedure entails risks of abnormal offspring higher than those associated with natural human reproduction."

Although EAB came out in favor of IVF research in 1979 in its recommendations to the Department of Health, Education and Welfare, the federal government is still dragging its feet and has given no money to researchers to support IVF. Pierre Soupart died on June 10, 1981, without receiving the grant he had applied for seven years earlier. Although the scientific community mourns the loss of this American IVF pioneer, his work lives on. Other doctors, including Anne Colston Wentz and James Daniell, have put into operation his dream of opening an IVF clinic at Vanderbilt. But all the test-tube baby clinics in the United States are feeling the effects of the lack of federal funds. In fact, the Joneses were only able to start their Norfolk clinic after receiving $25,000 from private individuals, including a wealthy Virginia woman who, earlier in her life, had become pregnant after medical treatments by Georgeanna Jones. (Write to your senators, representatives, and the current Secretary of Health and Human Services if you would like to press for the granting of federal monies to scientists for IVF research.)

• THE LAW AND IVF

The Ethics Advisory Board clarified many of the ethical issues encountered by the scientists and couples who are part of the IVF process. In the course of its deliberation, the board also focused attention on the state laws that appear to cover IVF. A final recommendation of the EAB was that a model law be drafted to clarify the rights of IVF offspring, parents, and those who participate in the process. Under the current crazy quilt of state laws, the legal rights of IVF participants are unclear. The board expressed concern not only about the legal status of IVF children but also warned about the current "lack of clarity regarding the legal responsibilities of those who utilize, support, or permit the use of such procedures."

State rather than federal law governs your relationship with your doctor. States, for example, have adopted statutes such as those dealing with doctor-patient communication and informed consent. In addition, state law governs family issues, such as the legitimacy of children, custody, and support, all of which have ramifications in the area of *in vitro* fertilization and the other new reproductive technologies. Even if a doctor or researcher were to receive federal funds, state laws would still apply to his or her work. Not all states have the same types of laws governing the doctor-patient relationship or families, so it is important to know the law of your specific state. To find out, consult a lawyer or your local American Civil Liberties Union branch.

As is true with all the new reproductive technologies, the legal status of *in vitro* fertilization is affected by two types of laws: (1) those that were on the books before the process was developed, yet by their language seem to cover it, and (2) those that were passed with the process specifically in mind.

Currently, IVF is not available in every state. In some states, doctors do not have the technical capabilities for or the interest in performing IVF. In other states, despite doctors who would like to offer the service and despite the presence of infertile couples who would like to participate in such programs, the doctors are fearful of opening IVF clinics because of laws that either seem to prohibit what they intend to do or would so restrict the doctors' actions that they do not feel they could adequately perform IVF within those constraints.

One type of law that was not generally intended to cover IVF but deters doctors from opening IVF clinics is a fetal research law. Nearly half the states have enacted laws restricting experimentation on fetuses. The impetus behind many of these laws was the legalization of abortion in the mid-1970s. Legislators felt that in order for people to maintain respect for human dignity, it was necessary to pass laws restricting or prohibiting doctors' experimentation on fetuses and on pregnant women who intended to abort. Of the 23 states with laws restricting experimentation on fetuses, 15 explicitly extend their coverage to research on embryos.

A minority of the laws restrict only research done at a time when an abortion is anticipated or subsequent to an abortion. Since *in vitro* fertilization does not involve an abortion, it is not covered by such provisions.

Laws that ban research on fetuses in a more general manner, however, might preclude the practice of *in vitro* fertilization. In Michigan, there can be no research on a live human embryo if its life or health may be jeopardized. A Maine law forbids experimentation on live fetuses, whether intrauterine or extrauterine. A Minnesota law forbids experimentation on a conceptus—including one conceived outside the body—unless the experiment protects its health or life, or scientific evidence has shown that sort of experiment to be harmless.

Doctors in states that ban research on embryos sometimes avoid offering IVF. They fear that their manipulation of the embryo in the petri dish or its implantation in the mother will be viewed as experimentation on a fetus. (After all, doctors have not yet perfected the IVF technique, so they often experiment with new approaches.) And since relatively little work on IVF has been done, the doctors may not be able to scientifically prove, to the satisfaction of a court, that what they are doing is beneficial to the fetus (rather than just beneficial to a couple who desperately want children). Fearful of being prosecuted as criminals, and of facing potential jail sentences or fines, some doctors in states with tight restrictions on fetal research have given up the idea of performing IVF at all.

Because of the fetal research laws, the contours of what a physician may do are being worked out on a state-by-state basis. For example, in Massachusetts in March 1983, the district attorney for the Boston area rendered an opinion that IVF would not violate the Massachusetts fetal research law if all the fertilized eggs were implanted in the woman.

The law's stance on fetal research was developed before the birth of Louise Brown and did not at all anticipate the test-tube baby technology. The actual achievement of IVF, though, triggered off a heated attack by various right-to-life groups, some of which have been pressuring state and local governments to ban IVF procedures. As was mentioned earlier, the Tidewater, Virginia, right-to-life group could not successfully stop the establishment of the Eastern Virginia Medical Clinic's IVF program. But right-to-life groups in Illinois successfully pressured the legislature to enact a law severely restricting the procedure in that state.

The Illinois law is the first in the country to single out IVF. It does so in a very strange way. It makes a doctor who fertilizes a woman's egg outside her body the custodian of that child for purposes of an 1877 child abuse act. The doctor is criminally liable if he or she endangers the life or health of the embryo. Thus the law does not prohibit *in vitro* fertilization directly, but raises so many concerns in the minds of Illinois doctors that virtually all have been unwilling to undertake the procedure.

How incongruous it is, though, to deal with the space-age issue of IVF by referring to an 1877 law! That is the problem: when lawmakers in the late 1800s designed that particular child protection law, they expected it to mean that a parent or guardian would provide sufficient food, clothing, and shelter so that a child would remain healthy. Doctors have no idea how judges will interpret this law to cover IVF. What must a doctor do to provide adequate care to a two-cell, four-cell, or eight-cell embryo? Can a doctor be prosecuted for child abuse if the district attorney believes the doctor should have provided different nutrients in the embryo's medium or should have stored the petri dish with the embryo at a different temperature? Will the doctor commit a crime if he or she discards an embryo that is not dividing properly?

The possibility that an Illinois doctor will have criminal liability in every action he or she undertakes with respect to the embryo is one reason the Illinois law impedes IVF in that state. Another reason is that the law grants custody to the doctor but never arranges for the parents to *regain* custody!

"The 'custody' imposed by the *in vitro* provision is open-ended," explains American Civil Liberties attorney Lois Lipton. "It does not terminate at implantation, birth, or any other determinate point in time. Under the law, the doctor appears to have custody even after the embryo is reimplanted. The doctor may even have custody after the child is born and matures into an adult! In addition, the *in vitro* provision implicitly denies custody to the natural parents."

If such a law had been in effect in England, Lesley and John Brown would have had no legal claim to Louise; instead, she would have belonged to Edwards and Steptoe.

If there is a law on the books in your state that appears to prohibit IVF, you have several choices. The first is to try to enter a program in another state. This has several disadvantages, not the least of which are the cost and inconvenience of travel each time you need a laparoscopy, implantation, or related procedure. In addition, the harsh restrictions on IVF in some states means a lengthy waiting list in states that do allow IVF. The Norfolk clinic, for example, currently has a backlog of about one thousand women wanting IVF. If American doctors make wider use of IVF for low sperm count as well as tubal problems, the lines will be even longer.

A sad side effect of the lengthy wait is that by the time your number is called, you may be too old to qualify for the program. In Houston, the cut-off age is thirty-eight. The wait may accentuate emotional problems as well. "By the time our program was operational, two years after we started taking applications, half of the first couples on our waiting list had separated or divorced," says Martin Quigley of the Houston clinic.

An alternative to forcing your way into a program in a distant state is battling your own state's restrictions head on. Like Lopata's patient who confronted the right-to-life group in the Australian hospital lobby, you can achieve a great deal by lobbying on behalf of a law that would allow IVF. It is amazing what you can accomplish by writing to or meeting with legislators and newspaper and broadcast reporters to let them know that those who wish to use IVF are nice normal couples who would make good parents and who wish to privately undertake with their doctors a medical procedure to allow them to bear children. Expressing your heart-felt desire for children would help to challenge their misperception that IVF involves mad scientists who would plunge us into a Brave New World. Your efforts will be even more forceful if you involve your local Resolve group or other patients in your doctor's infertility practice, even if these other infertile couples have different physical problems and are not candidates for IVF. Couples who are considering childbearing by any of the new reproductive technologies should unite in their efforts to contact lawmakers, since many legal changes are necessary before IVF, artificial insemination, surrogate motherhood, or other new reproductive technologies become viable options throughout the entire United States.

In addition to promoting the benefits of the New Conceptions through lobbying, you might wish to take an even more assertive step and litigate. An Illinois couple joined with their doctor, Aaron Lifchez, to file suit in an Illinois federal court challenging the Illinois IVF law. The couple, who wished to remain anonymous, called themselves Mary and John Smith on the legal papers. They brought the suit as a class action, on behalf of all infertile couples who might benefit from IVF. In this way, if they win, they will not just win the narrow right for Lifchez to fertilize Mary's egg with John's sperm. Rather, they will gain a court order declaring the law itself unconstitutional and allowing any couple who wants IVF in Illinois to undergo the procedure with their individual doctors.

Mary and John have been married for seven years and have two adopted children. For them, IVF represents the only way that they will be able to conceive a child. Mary's tubes were damaged nineteen years ago when her appendix ruptured when she was fifteen. She underwent a number of corrective operations on her tubes, but the original damage was just too great. Lifchez advised the couple that IVF was their only available method of conception.

The chances of Mary being accepted into an IVF program in another state are very slim. She was thirty-four years old when she filed suit and would be too old to qualify for some programs if she were on a waiting list for more than a year. (Besides, Mary and

John have confidence in their own doctor and know that the medical center at which he practices has the medical and physical capabilities to commence an IVF program.) The only reason Dr. Lifchez was unwilling to offer *in vitro* fertilization to the Smiths was his fear of being prosecuted for child abuse.

So, with the help of Lipton, Frances J. Krasnow of the Chicago law firm of Fohrman, Lurie, Sklar & Simon, Ltd., and myself, the Smiths and Lifchez are challenging the Illinois law. The premise of our suit—and of any lawsuit you may bring to challenge your state's restrictions on IVF—is as follows: just because a state law is on the books does not mean that it can withstand a challenge in court. The highest law in this country is the Constitution, so in instances where a fundamental constitutional right conflicts with a state law, the latter will be struck down unless the state can prove that it has a compelling need for such a law and that the law is drafted narrowly enough to just take care of that need without infringing on other legitimate activities.

The fundamental constitutional right on which proponents of new reproductive technologies should try to rely is that of privacy. In the past, that right has served as the basis for striking down a number of laws that interfered with couples' decisions about childbearing. In 1965, the U.S. Supreme Court struck down a law forbidding the use of contraceptives because it infringed on the right of marital privacy. U.S. Supreme Court Justice Goldberg, concurring in the decision, noted that "the entire fabric of the Constitution and the purposes that clearly underlie its specific guarantees demonstrate that the rights of marital privacy and to marry and raise a family are of similar order and magnitude as the fundamental rights specifically protected." Another U.S. Supreme Court case found that the right to procreate is "one of the basic civil rights of man. Marriage and procreation are fundamental to the very existence and survival of the race."

More recently, the U.S. Supreme Court wrote: "If the right of privacy means anything, it is the right of the individual, married or single, to be free of unwarranted govermental intrusion into matters so fundamentally affecting a person as the decision whether to bear or beget a child."

These cases establish the right of a couple, as part of their privacy right, to decide whether or not they will bear a child. In lawsuits about the new reproductive technologies, the question will be how far does that right go? There is no question that a married couple has a right to determine whether and when to bear a child through intercourse. Does a couple also have the right to decide *how* they would like to bear a child, even if it entails involving medical technology such as IVF in the process? It would certainly seem that the right to marital privacy should cover such a situation, and that is exactly what we argued for the Smiths in the Illinois case.

"While the legislature apparently views *in vitro* fertilization as a crime," we wrote in our brief, "to many childless couples it is seen as a possible miracle." We asserted that "the *in vitro* provision implicates and eviscerates both marital privacy and the individual privacy right to make and effectuate childbearing decisions. Procreation is universally recognized by every culture and religion as a fundamental element of the institution of marriage. For many married couples it is the essence of family. The desire to produce one's own offspring is, for most couples, as primary as the need to eat or sleep." Because of the constitutional protection given the extremely important childbearing decision, we argued that the Illinois law interfering with that decision should be declared unconstitutional.

Other lawyers agree that a statute prohibiting IVF is unconstitutional. "Such a law would certainly infringe a fundamental interest of infertile women—their right to bear children," wrote Philip Reilly, who holds both a medical and a law degree. "It might also infringe the first amendment rights of the clinical researchers by improperly restricting their freedom of inquiry." The same argument could be made against *any* type of law that inhibits IVF even if the law was designed for some other purpose, such as the prohibition of fetal research. If a fundamental privacy right to choose how to bear a child is recognized by the courts, then even laws adopted for other valid purposes will need to be amended so that they are narrow enough to cover just that purpose and not infringe upon IVF.

After we filed suit challenging the Illinois *in vitro* law, the Illinois Attorney General and the State's Attorney for Cook County rendered an opinion that any physician who undertakes IVF would not violate the law as long as the physician refrained "from wilfully endangering or injuring" the embryo during the preimplantation period. They said that if an embryo was terminated because it was defective, that action would be interpreted as a lawful pregnancy termination on the part of the physician. This opinion set the stage for *in vitro* fertilization to go forward in Illinois.

If you are worried about laws that prohibit IVF, pay close attention to what is happening in the U.S. Congress. Federal lawmakers are considering passing the Human Life Bill, which would give an embryo full legal rights from the moment of conception. John D. Gorby, director of the Legal Defense Fund of Americans United for Life, and professor at John Marshall Law School in Chicago, has rendered a legal opinion that passage of the Human Life Bill would prohibit the test-tube baby process.

Not all the laws applicable to IVF erect barriers to the process. An *in vitro* fertilization law was enacted in Pennsylvania to monitor the procedure. The law provides that anyone conducting IVF must file quarterly reports with the Department of Health describing the events. Other existing legal doctrines give rights to couples undergoing the procedure. For example, certain laws give couples the right to information. A doctor is legally required to obtain the couple's informed consent before beginning IVF; to do so, he or she must explain to the couple, in understandable terms, the steps that will be undertaken and the risks of each of these steps. Couples also have legal rights to their eggs, sperm, or embryo even when they are in the lab, and already one lawsuit established a couple's right to collect damages when someone tries to thwart their *in vitro* fertilization.

In 1973, Doris and John Del Zio, a Florida couple, became the first couple in the United States to attempt IVF. Doris' New York City infertility specialist, Dr. William Sweeney, had tried three times to repair her fallopian tubes, but she had not managed to successfully carry a pregnancy to term. Sweeney felt additional surgery would be of no benefit, so he decided to suggest a procedure that was only a glimmer in the eyes of researchers in 1973—*in vitro* fertilization. At that time, although Steptoe and Edwards had reported in the scientific literature that they had fertilized human eggs outside of the body, there apparently had been no successful reimplantations. The possibility of Del Zio giving birth through IVF was very speculative indeed.

Sweeney asked Dr. Landrum Shettles of Manhattan's Columbia Presbyterian Medical Center to aid in the procedure. Geographical distance made their collaboration difficult, though; the hospital where Sweeney would remove the egg was on East 70th Street in New York, while Shettles' laboratory was on West 168th Street. Nevertheless, on September 12, 1973, Sweeney removed an egg from Doris Del Zio via laparoscopy, putting it in a sterile container with protective packing. John Del Zio then carried the package across town in a taxi to the Columbia Presbyterian laboratory. There, after the addition of John Del Zio's sperm, the culture medium with the egg was placed in an incubator to develop for three days before an attempt at implantation in Doris Del Zio.

The day after the laparoscopy, however, Shettles was ordered to the office of his boss, Dr. Raymond Vande Wiele, the chairman of the Department of Obstetrics and Gynecology at Columbia Presbyterian Hospital and Medical Center. Vande Wiele was furious that Shettles had attempted this sort of experiment without following the procedure of seeking the institution's permission. Vande Wiele noted that research should have been undertaken with monkeys before subjecting a human to the procedure; he felt that it was unethical and immoral to carry on this work with Doris Del Zio. Later Vande Wiele claimed that he had been worried that the contents of the petri dish were contaminated and he did not want to see Del Zio risk infection or even death if it were implanted in her uterus.

Vande Wiele did more than vent his wrath on Shettles. He had taken the responsibility for ending the experiment entirely. Atop Vande Wiele's desk stood the Del Zio container. He had removed it from the incubator and opened it, thus dashing completely their hopes of giving birth to a child through *in vitro* fertilization.

At that moment, Doris Del Zio was still hospitalized, recovering from the laparoscopy. When the news reached her, she sank into a profound depression. She had lost her last chance to become a mother; Sweeney had told her that her tubes were so badly damaged he could not attempt to remove another egg. A year later, she and her husband filed suit against Columbia Presbyterian Medical Center, Columbia University, and Raymond Vande Wiele.

In 1974, when the suit was filed, there seemed to be little chance of its success. The whole process of IVF seemed like something out of a science fiction story, so it would be difficult to convince a jury that the Del Zios had indeed lost a chance to become parents. The wheels of justice grind slowly, however, and it was July 17, 1978, before a trial began in the Del Zio case.

In a remarkable bit of timing, nine days into the five-week trial, headlines screamed forth the news of Louise Brown's birth in England. A defense attorney tried to prevent the jury from being influenced by the success across the ocean. He said scornfully that Shettles' procedure was as distinct from the English technique as "a Model T Ford is from a Porsche."

Perhaps because they now believed that a test-tube birth was possible, the jurors awarded Doris Del Zio $50,000 for her mental anguish. The jury decided that the defendant's conduct was so extreme, outrageous, and shocking that it exceeded all reasonable bounds of decency. (In an interesting twist to this particular case, Vande Wiele has now started an *in vitro* clinic at Columbia.)

• *THE IVF CHILD*

While the ethical and legal furor surrounding petri dish procreation continues, couples around the world are finding their dreams of childbearing fulfilled by *in vitro* fertilization. Quietly and without fanfare, hundreds of test-tube babies have joined the ranks of Louise Brown and Elizabeth Carr. In 1984, a thousand women will be pregnant through *in vitro* fertilization. Paul Ramsey, a Protestant theologian at Princeton University, speculates that a test-tube baby could suffer from damage to his or her self-image because of media fanfare surrounding the process. As a growing number of children are nurtured into life in a petri dish, however, the chances of stigma from notoriety will diminish. After all, every child they bear in any manner is unique and special to a previously infertile couple.

"Does it worry you that she may carry the label 'test-tube baby'?" PBS reporter Peter Williams asked Judy Carr.

"No, it doesn't worry me," she replied. "I think this will all die down and she'll just be our Elizabeth."

7 ❧ Artificial Insemination

A week before Brenda and Tom's wedding, they received devastating news. Tom was sterile. He had undergone a sperm count and there were zero sperm in it. "Should we still get married?" he asked Brenda. She did not know what to say. She loved Tom, but, she thought to herself, one of the reasons I wanted to get married was to have babies.

Brenda did not want to upset Tom even further, though. So she went through with the marriage, pretending to be the happy, carefree bride. Inside, she felt as if a part of her had died.

"People feel they will fall in love, get married, and have children," she explains. "It's a piece of life we expect to happen and we were robbed of that."

The conflict between the surface happiness of the newlyweds and their inner turmoil continued for three years. Neighbors' casual questions of "When are you going to have a baby?" would pierce them like a knife.

During that period. Brenda brought up the idea of artificial insemination, but Tom continually refused. They called adoption agencies but were put off by various regulations: they had not been married long enough, there was a conflict in their religions, or the agency did not approve of Brenda working. Brenda again asked Tom to consider artificial insemination.

"When he didn't want to go ahead with artificial insemination, I felt that he was rejecting me," Brenda recalls. "We had discussed the possibility of having children for years before we got married.

Now I worried that he had found something wrong with me and thought I wouldn't be a good parent."

Finally, after three years of biting her tongue on the question, Brenda asked, "Why don't you want me to have a baby?"

"It turned out he had opposed AID because he was misinformed," Brenda remarks. "He thought anybody who walked off the street could be a donor. He thought the donor would be a Skid Row bum and that the child would be diseased."

When Tom learned that most donors were medical students who were screened by the doctor, he agreed to the procedure. The conversation with the doctor raised more questions than it answered for Brenda.

"I had about thirty questions," she says, "but I was afraid to ask them. The one attempt I made was brushed off. They had said they would use frozen sperm and I asked what that was. A nurse said it was sperm that had to be defrosted and then she disappeared out the door."

The first attempt at insemination succeeded. Brenda, however, spent the entire pregnancy worrying. Since the qualities of frozen sperm had not been explained to her, she confesses, "I spent nine months fearful that the freezing had damaged the sperm and that the child would be defective."

A baby girl was born, perfectly healthy and normal. She is now nine years old and still brings wonder and joy to Tom and Brenda (not their real names), who view themselves as equal parents.

Today, a decade after Brenda and Tom agreed to artificial insemination, the practice is growing. More importantly, information and counseling are readily available for couples so that they can undergo the procedure without the fears and doubts that Brenda and Tom experienced.

Artificial insemination by donor (AID) is used when the man is infertile. Currently, about ten thousand to twenty thousand AID children are born in the United States each year. The process has a 57 percent national success rate and is felt by many to offer a favorable alternative to adoption.

"I explain to couples that donor insemination is like adopting sperm," says Richard Amelar, who with his partner, Lawrence Dubin, conducts a New York City urology practice concentrating exclusively on male infertility.

Traditional adoption is becoming more difficult, with waits of three to five years. Artificial insemination generally achieves a pregnancy within three to five menstrual cycles. There is not the same red tape and microscopic probing into your life as in adopting a child, and women who may not be eligible to adopt—such as women over age forty—can become mothers through AID. Unlike adoption, there is no threat of the appearance of the mother who gave up the child. There is also little threat of the biological father appearing. Donors are not told whether a pregnancy has actually been achieved with their sperm, so it is unlikely a donor could form an attachment to the child and seek it out.

Artificial insemination offers other advantages. "I could experience Mary Lou being pregnant," comments one AID father. AID allows the couple and growing fetus to establish themselves as a family unit and to bond at an earlier stage. The husband can listen to the child's heartbeat through a stethoscope and feel the baby kick. He can participate in the delivery. After the birth, the wife can breast-feed.

The couple can also do more to ensure the health of the child. "When you adopt a child, you generally know nothing about the father and you don't know if the mother took drugs or failed to look after herself during this pregnancy that she didn't want," observes Amelar. With AID, the couple can provide a healthy prenatal environment for the child. "And the usual cost of donor insemination is several hundred dollars, not several thousands of dollars (as in adoption)" Amelar adds.

Some couples also like their children to resemble each other, which is unlikely in the case of adoption. With artificial insemination, all the children will have a genetic bond and resemblance to the mother. Couples can request that the sperm of a particular donor be frozen so that they can space their AID pregnancies, yet use the same donor. In this way, the physical similarity between the children will be even greater.

"AID is not for everyone," warns Los Angeles psychotherapist Annette Baran. The couple's initial feelings about the man's infertility must be worked through before AID is started.

"The couple is ready for insemination only if they will view the child not as a product of AID, but as a product of the marriage," states Betty Orlandino, founder of Human Relations Counseling, which offers information and psychological support to AID couples.

• *WHEN SHOULD AID BE USED?*

Artificial insemination by a donor is suggested for infertile couples in which the husband cannot impregnate his wife because of impotence, azoospermia (the absence of sperm), or oligospermia (a low sperm count). Up to 7 percent of couples requesting AID, however, are fertile; they choose it because they have Rh incompatibilities or the husband does not want to pass on a potential genetic defect such as the inheritable forms of Down's syndrome, blindness, Huntington's chorea, or Tay-Sachs disease. Since genetic testing is not yet available for every potential hereditary disorder, some men who merely suspect they carry a troublesome gene are forced to decide whether to go ahead with AID just to be sure.

"We had one man request AID because there was a lot of bone cancer in his family," remarks Steve Broder, supervisor of the Southern California Cryobank in Los Angeles. "He didn't know if he was a carrier, but he didn't want to take a chance."

As evidence mounts that exposure to radiation or particular chemicals or drugs causes chromosomal defects to offspring, some men consider AID when they have been in contact with workplace toxins or are undergoing chemotherapy. Military men who were exposed to Agent Orange and fear its effect on their offspring have already sought AID.

AID may also be a logical solution to some combined fertility problems, such as when the wife develops antibodies to the husband's sperm (so long as she does not have antibodies to all male sperm) or when medical treatments to enhance fertility do not work or are impractical within time constraints. Richard Amelar recommends AID when there is long-standing unexplained infertility in a couple who have exhausted all other treatments.

"The age of the woman is important," says Amelar. "I'll suggest AID if the woman is near the end of her reproductive years and the husband has poor quality semen. In this way, the couple will not miss the opportunity to have a child. The husband can continue to be treated and if he improves, the couple can then have a second child fathered by the husband."

If you are considering AID, it is important to make sure that the procedure is really necessary. According to one English infertility specialist, increased knowledge about the availability of AID has led to the referral of many patients for the procedure prior to an adequate investigation. He found that in one year alone 15 percent of the patients referred to him (65 out of 461 men) did not really need AID. Another clinician found that 25 percent of the men referred to him for AID had treatable disorders. These AID practitioners found that a number of male patients had undiagnosed varicoceles, varicose veins in the spermatic cord that interfere with sperm production. The varicoceles could be corrected with surgery, resulting in a 40 to 60 percent chance of achieving a pregnancy and eliminating the need for AID.

If you are considering AID because of impotence, you should be aware that great strides are being made in its treatment. Impotence frequently has a physical cause. Nerve and blood vessel disease or hormonal abnormalities cause one third of all impotence. Among the latest and sometimes controversial treatments to restore sexual potency are hormonal therapy, surgical implants, and an experimental blood vessel bypass operation. In addition, sometimes a prescribed drug causes the problem and the man can be cured by changing medications. You might want to find out more about the treatment of impotence before proceeding directly to AID.

If azoospermia is the problem, perhaps you should consider a testicular biopsy. Since the interpretation of such a test is complicated, it is worth having done only if it is performed by an expert. By taking an extremely thin slice from a man's testicle, a well-trained expert can discover whether sperm is being produced. If none is produced, then there is absolutely no chance the man can biologically father a child. If the azoospermic man is *producing* sperm, but they are just not getting out into the semen, the doctor can investigate further and correct by surgery any blockage that is impeding the sperm from making its way into the ejaculate.

Oligospermia, another common reason for AID, is also the most problematic. Some men are told to undergo AID on the basis of a single sperm count. You should refuse to even consider AID under those circumstances. As you know, many environmental and internal forces can affect a sperm count. If a man had the flu three months earlier or if he has increased the temperature of his testicles by wearing tight underwear, taking hot baths, or even driving long distances, the count will register low, even if the man is really fertile. Before making an AID referral, a competent doctor will order additional sperm counts with sufficient time in between and counsel the man about how changes in his activities may help increase his sperm count.

Many men wonder how low a sperm count must be in order for AID to considered. The procedure is recommended for couples in which the man has a sperm count under twenty million per cubic centimeter (cc). That does not mean that if your count is less than that you should immediately try AID. Plenty of men who have impregnated their wives have sperm counts of under twenty million per cc. In fact, a study of over two thousand fertile men by Emil Steinberger of the University of Texas found that 23 percent of these *fertile* men (who had all achieved pregnancies) had counts of under twenty million per cc and 11.7 percent had counts of under ten million.

Ironically, one doctor turned away a potential sperm donor because he had a count of only ten million per cc, which classified him as infertile. The man told his wife she could stop using contraceptives. A month later, she was pregnant. Another doctor reported on five men with counts below one million per cc who also stopped contraception. Four of the five became fathers!

Because the sperm count is an imperfect predictor of a man's ability to impregnate a woman, couples should not rush into AID even if repeated sperm counts register low. They still have a good chance of creating a child naturally, and should make every effort to enhance that chance. It takes two to create a pregnancy and sometimes subfertility in one spouse can be "treated" by enhancing fertility in the other spouse.

If a man is oligospermic, his wife should be investigated (and treated if necessary) for such things as hostile cervical mucus and ovulating irregularities. In that way, the few sperm the oligospermic man has will have an easier time traveling through the woman's reproductive tract and fertilizing an egg.

Artificial insemination by husband (AIH), in which the husband's semen is collected and then injected into the wife's vagina near her cervix or in her cervical canal, is another way to give sperm a boost and enhance the chances of pregnancy. Men with counts as low as five to ten million per cc have a 50 percent chance of achieving pregnancy if full treatment is given the wife.

Even after treatment of both spouses and extended attempts at natural pregnancy, there will be some couples who have not conceived. Before turning to AID, though, you might consider the possibility of *in vitro* fertilization. IVF offers hope to low sperm count men because many fewer sperm are needed to ensure fertilization of an egg *in vitro* than in regular intercourse or AIH. The Houston IVF clinic run by Martin Quigley, for example, accepts couples in which the man has a sperm count—in the *total* ejaculate—of at least two million. That means that if the man ejaculates, say, five cubic centimeters of semen, his count per centimeter need only be 400,000.

For some couples—and clearly for the azoospermic, who produces *no* sperm that could be used in IVF or AIH—AID will be the treatment of choice. But even when AID seems right for physical reasons, the time to go forward depends on emotional considerations as well. "I don't think anyone who learns of his infertility for the first time is able to make a judgment at that point regarding donor insemination," suggests Amelar. "The man must have time to recover from the shock of learning about his infertility."

A time lag before AID is mandatory for couples in France. "Your first consultation for AID does not happen until six months after you make your phone call to the clinic and the insemination does not take place until a year later," reports Simone Novaes, a sociologist who researches artificial insemination for France's National Center for Scientific Research.

In Denmark, a couple is required to wait three months to a year for AID, depending on their ages. About 20 percent of the couples decide during that time that they do not want to proceed with AID.

• *THE HISTORY OF THE AID PROCEDURE*

The actual AID procedure has been used for nearly a century in this country. In 1884, Dr. William Pancoast, a medical school professor, was approached by a wealthy Philadelphia couple who had been trying unsuccessfully to have a child. The cause of the problem seemed to be with the husband, so Pancoast looked for someone to donate semen to be injected into the wife's womb. He asked the best-looking member of his class to volunteer, and since the injection was done under anesthesia, Pancoast performed the AID without the knowledge of either the husband or the wife.

The baby's birth, though, gave the doctor some pause. The infant so resembled the student that Pancoast felt obliged to explain to the husband what he had done. The rich Philadelphian, happy to have a child, was delighted by the good doctor's creativity. He asked only that his wife never be told the origin of the child.

Today, it would be illegal for a doctor to perform AID on a woman without her consent. However, the secrecy surrounding AID has in many ways continued. Some doctors are reluctant to disclose to couples important aspects of the procedure. To ensure that you have the greatest chance of producing a healthy baby within a reasonable period of treatment, you should exercise your right to medical information and ask your doctor to explain his or her method of donor selection, whether fresh or frozen semen will be used, and what attempts will be made to pinpoint the time of ovulation.

• *DONOR SELECTION*

Although you may want to ask your doctor many questions about donor selection, two key questions that should not be forgotten are: What do you do to ensure that the donor does not transmit a genetic or venereal disease? How many pregnancies do you allow any one donor to create?

Most doctors insist that the couple have blind faith in the doctor's choice of a donor. But a large-scale study undertaken by two geneticists, Martin Curie-Cohen and Lesleigh Luttrell, and an endocrinologist, Sander Shapiro, of the University of Wisconsin, and published in the March 15, 1979 *New England Journal of Medicine* indicates that such faith may be misplaced. Many doctors did little screening of donors, which put sperm recipients at risk for contracting venereal disease or giving birth to a child with a genetic defect.

Imagine your distress if you were artificially inseminated in your doctor's office, but instead of getting a child you ended up getting gonorrhea! It has happened. In fact, a wide range of viruses and bacteria have been transmitted through AID. Even freezing the sperm does not help; infections such as gonorrhea are known to live at least two years in frozen semem. Infections can cause tubal problems, potentially making the woman infertile and thus totally dashing the couple's hope of ever having a child who is genetically related to one of them. Some doctors who use frozen sperm add the antibiotics penicillin and streptomycin to semen before they freeze it, but this has no demonstrated benefit since the antibiotic loses its ability to fight once the mixture is frozen. Plus the woman might have an allergic reaction to the antibiotic.

The problem of AID-caused infections has been recognized by two professional organizations. The American Fertility Society (AFS), the professional association of infertility specialists, publishes guidelines covering all aspects of AID. The guidelines recommend that a sperm specimen from a donor be cultured for gonorrhea *before* the anticipated need for the donor. Even if the donor is initially infection-free, subsequent specimens should be cultured if there are white cells present, indicating an infection.

The American Association of Tissue Banks (AATB) is an association of the professionals and scientists involved with cell, tissue, and organ banking. The AATB's Reproductive Council is concerned with sperm banking and has drafted standards to ensure a minimum level of donor screening. These standards suggest that each sperm sample from the donor be tested for gonorrhea, with periodic analysis of the donor's blood for syphillis and hepatitis.

In addition to the potential for infections that may put the recipient woman at risk, the donor may pass on a genetic defect that would be harmful or even fatal to the AID child. To help guard against that possibility, the American Fertility Society suggests that doctors investigate the donor's family history and reject prospective donors with a family history of mental retardation, neurologic disorders, unexplained deaths under age thirty, or significant congenital defects. The AFS also suggests that the Tay-Sachs trait should be screened for in Jewish donors and sickle cell trait should be screened for in black donors. Laboratory tests should be performed to ensure that the donor and recipient have compatible Rh factors.

The AATB standards are even more detailed, listing nineteen types of disorders that should prohibit men from being sperm donors and describing tests that could be performed to determine whether the potential donor might be a carrier of these disorders. These guidelines also suggest that when the family history of a donor is taken, the professional should consider contacting the physicians of the family members discussed to document the health status or cause of death of that person. According to the standards, "A report of any condition in a prospective donor's family history which might put him at risk of more than one percent for producing a child with a birth defect and/or a genetic disease would disqualify him as a donor." The AATB also suggests rejecting donors who have been alcohol or drug abusers or who have worked at a job with any significant risk of radiation or chemical exposure.

The AFS and AATB guidelines provide a solid basis for avoiding genetic mishaps with AID. Unfortunately, the majority of AID practitioners apparently do not follow these standards. Curie-

Cohen, Luttrell, and Shapiro surveyed 379 AID practitioners, most of whom were members of the American Fertility Society. These 379 doctors had been responsible for 3,576 AID births in 1977. Although 96 percent took some form of family history from the donors, this "history" often consisted of just asking the donor to indicate family health problems on a short list of common diseases. The doctors rarely had any training in genetics. Only 29 percent performed blood tests on donors, and most of these tests were for communicable diseases (such as venereal diseases), not genetic disorders. Although 94.7 percent of the doctors assured researchers that they would reject a donor who carried the Tay-Sachs trait, less than 1 percent tested donors for the trait. Although 92 percent said they would reject a potential donor with a translocation or trisomy (genetic defects that show up on karyotypes), only 12.5 percent bothered to learn what the potential donor's karyotype actually was. The University of Wisconsin researchers concluded, "The screening of donors for genetic diseases is inadequate."

At conferences and in private interviews, doctors offer various rationales for the superficiality of their screening. Some say that they rely on medical students as donors and trust that students would not lie about being healthy when they were not. Even if medical students (who are paid for their sperm donation) are able to recognize that they have an infection and are trustworthy enough not to donate sperm at that time, the medical student's self-report should not be relied on to disclose genetic disorders. There are over twenty-five hundred identifiable genetic disorders and even the well-intentioned student donor may not realize he is a carrier. "It is sobering," state the AATB guidelines," to realize that about one in 150 in the population has a chromosomal abnormality."

For example, a student donor may not be aware that he is a carrier of Tay-Sachs. The issue may never have come up in the donor's life. If the donor is single and has no children, he would have had no opportunity to learn that he has the Tay-Sachs trait. If he is married to a woman who herself does not carry the trait, their children would have been born normal and the possibility of

Tay-Sachs may never have entered his consciousness. Even if he and his wife are carriers, they have a 75 percent chance of producing a healthy child.

A study of 168 donor applicants at the University of North Carolina School of Medicine demonstrated the problem of relying on donors' self-reports. According to the researchers, "the majority of donors having a positive family history [of a genetic disorder] did not recognize the condition as being genetic, even if the individual had had medical training."

The inadequacy of donor screening has already had fatal results. A couple who had tried unsuccessfully to conceive a child for five years turned to AID. The wife gave birth to a daughter, who after a year of health, began to lose her vision and coordination. At two years, she began to have seizures, which, by two and a half years occurred every five to ten minutes.

Doctors at Columbia University College of Physicians and Surgeons (where the girl was brought for treatment) tried to unravel what had happened. They speculated that the donor was a carrier of Tay-Sachs. Perhaps the inseminating doctors did not bother to screen the donor for Tay-Sachs because the recipient was of Italian extraction, not Jewish. The doctor may have felt that, even if the donor was a carrier, there would be little chance that the woman would be a carrier, too. Tragically, though, the woman carried a gene that was similar enough to the Tay-Sachs trait to create a devastatingly ill child.

Another couple sought AID because the husband suffered from oligospermia. The doctor picked a donor who had produced four healthy children. An AID daughter was born who became ill at three months and died before her second birthday. The couple wanted another child, so they used AID again. The doctor used the same donor and the couple had to relive that nightmare. A son was born, and at age two months he fell prey to the same illness and died shortly thereafter.

Two University of Michigan Medical School professors who described this family's situation in a report in the *New England Journal of Medicine* issued the following warning: "These cases illustrate the necessity of extreme caution in using sperm from the same donor for artificial insemination when one child thus conceived is afflicted with an unknown disorder, even if the problem is presumed not to have been inherited." Yet many doctors do not keep records of which donors were used for which pregnancies. Seventy percent of the doctors surveyed by Curie-Cohen, Luttrell, and Shapiro said they kept no donor records. One eminent specialist reveals: "Six months after the child's birth, we eliminate the donor's records." Yet some genetic defects will not occur until later in the child's life.

Moreover, some doctors inseminate the woman with the sperm of several donors in the same cycle to deliberately confuse the issue of paternity (and thus protect the men) by making it difficult to determine which donor was actually responsible for the pregnancy. Such practices make it hard to identify the donor who has caused a genetic defect and thus exclude him from other inseminations.

Some doctors justify a haphazard approach to screening and recordkeeping by saying that a woman who conceives in the natural manner runs the risk of infection or a genetically defective child, so AID recipients should not expect less risk.

But a couple who chooses AID *does* deserve more. At an English conference on artificial insemination, obstetrician D. Ellis was flabbergasted that doctors were even suggesting the AID should not offer higher quality controls than a quick fling with a stranger.

"Then why operate AID at all?" asked Ellis, suggesting that if doctors were so lax, the patient might as well get pregnant by anyone. "If we are offering a service then we have to offer a service which says that the sperm are good sperm, that the patient will become pregnant after two or three tries, that she will have as normal a baby as we can manage, that she will not get infected, that it will be totally anonymous, that there will be no contact with the donor but that we will know that he is efficient."

Theologian G. R. Dunstan agreed, stating that doctors providing AID should use "higher criteria than those provided by natural random forces." After all, a growing number of women undergo AID precisely because they want to avoid "random forces"—the potential genetic problems that could be passed on by their husbands.

At that same English conference, one speaker expressed his belief that donors should not be required to undergo physical examinations or blood tests to determine their chromosomal makeup because such tests would be bothersome.

"I am outraged by the suggestion that we should perhaps avoid making a careful clinical examination of a donor because he may find it unpleasant," said Swedish physiologist R. Elliasson. "Why do we not do away with the regulations that the pharmaceutical industry finds unpleasant?"

Some doctors allow carriers of a recessive genetic defect to donate sperm so long as the recipient does not have that defect. Other doctors oppose that approach. They point out that a conception between a carrier and noncarrier will not lead to a child who suffers from the disease (and thus would seem to meet the couple's desire for a healthy baby). However, although healthy, that baby will have a 50 percent chance of being a carrier of the disease, and thus of passing it on to his or her own child if he or she marries another carrier. They advocate rejecting as donors all carriers of serious defects.

It is ironic that the screening of donor sperm for human AID is much less stringent than that of bull sperm in the cattle industry. For example, bull sperm is frozen and not used for at least a month after it is collected so that sufficient tests can be performed and checkups can be done on the animal to ensure that it was not carrying an undetected infection at the time it gave the sperm. Records are maintained tracing the health of all offspring of the donor, and the laboratory staff undergo periodic tests of their health to limit the risk of transmitting viruses or bacteria to the samples. According to a number of doctors, similar standards of excellence should be adopted by practitioners of human AID.

Along those lines, the Judicial Council of the American Medical Association in May 1983, issued an opinion stating:

> Physicians have an ethical responsibility to use the utmost caution and scientifically available screening techniques in the selection of donors for use in artificial insemination.

Relying only upon the verbal representations of donors as to their health, without any medical screening, is precarious. The donor should be screened for genetic defects, inheritable and infectious disease, Rh factor incompatibility and other disorders that may affect the fetus. When the physician is not equipped to fulfill these responsibilities, the services of a skilled medical geneticist or other appropriate specialist should be sought.

Doctors assert that screening all donors is too costly a proposition. But many couples would be willing to pay $35 for a Tay-Sachs test of the donor or even $250 for a complete karyotyping. After all, they are already paying an average of $720 for the sperm alone over the course of several months of AID attempts.

One doctor in the audience of a medical meeting urged participants to give couples more options regarding the testing of donors. "A good rule of thumb for the type of testing you should offer the patient is 'What would I do if I were sitting on the other side of the desk,'" he declared. "I would want a complete chromosomal analysis."

The AATB standards state that the decision to do karyotyping on a donor should ultimately be up to the infertile couple. But many couples are not informed of the possibility of requesting donor screening of any type. According to a study by Mark Frankel, project director of the Center for the Study of Ethics in the Professions at the Illinois Institute of Technology, "There is little evidence to suggest that the prospective recipients of donor semen are presented with the full range of alternatives and given the option of requesting that certain tests be performed." Clearly, you may have to take the initiative and question your doctor specifically and at length about the type of screening you would like performed on your donor.

• *AGE SCREENING AND EXTENT OF SPERM USE*

Once an AID practitioner has a pool of donors whose health has been established according to existing tests, other selection criteria, such as the age of the donor, become important. The Repository for Germinal Choice, the bank established in California for sperm of Nobel Prize winners, accepts sperm from donors who are in their seventies. However, the guidelines of both the AFS and the AATB suggest that no man over the age of thirty-five be allowed to donate, since genetic abnormalities in children increase as the age of the genetic father increases. For example, contrary to popular misconceptions, an older father (even without an older mother) has an increased chance of conceiving a Down's syndrome child. Also, there is evidence that sperm loses its fertilizing capability beginning in early adulthood, leading some experts to suggest a maximum donor age as low as twenty-five.

Another critical question concerns how many children a donor will be allowed to father. The study by Curie-Cohen, Luttrell, and Shapiro found that most doctors used each donor for up to six pregnancies. Six percent used the same donor for fifteen or more. One doctor continued using a single donor for fifty pregnancies. It is biologically possible for a single donor's sperm to father as many as twenty thousand AID children in one year.

While doctors like to continue using donors of proven fertility, widespread use of a single donor in a limited geographical area could lead to unwitting incest if children of the same donor grow up and marry each other. The possibility is remote, but in Tel Aviv, a marriage has already occurred between two AID children fathered by the same donor. In the United States a similar marriage was stopped by a doctor who revealed to the couple their genetic link. Thus, it seems wise to put some limit on the number of donor pregnancies a man is allowed to initiate.

Because of the uncertainties of using the sperm from an anonymous donor, some couples will ask that the doctor do the insemination with sperm from a man who is known to them. "There is a certain logic in using the father or brother of the husband," obstetrician D. N. Joyce conceded. "However, the possibility of subsequent emotional problems of a sexual nature, or in relation to ownership of the child, far outweigh any potential advantages. I could not agree to such an agreement, although apparently successful cases of family donors have been recorded."

In one southern state, there were two identical twin brothers, one fertile and one sterile. They approached a medical center so that the fertile one could serve as a stand-in for his twin through artificial insemination. At the last minute, though, they changed their minds. The wife of the fertile one did not want her sister-in-law raising her husband's children!

• *UNREALISTIC PROMISES*

Although couples have not been given much choice about the age, number of offspring, or testing done on the donor, couples are often given a form and told to list the physical and personality traits they would like in the donor. Some practices allow people to indicte whether they want someone who is athletic, musically inclined, has dimples, or is a member of a certain religion. Yet the doctors apparently do not inform couples about the poor chance of meeting their carefully thought-out request.

Even at the large commercial sperm banks, the supply of donors is limited. At the Southern California Cryobank, for instance, the entire line of frozen sperm has been obtained from just twenty-five donors. Private practitioners using fresh sperm have even fewer donor choices available even though they, too, may encourage couples to describe exactly what they want. In addition, even if a practitioner has available sperm from a donor possessing the desired traits, there is no evidence that many traits listed are inheritable.

Although specific personality traits and talent are not deliverable through AID, doctors can match physical characteristics of the donor to that of the husband. In some situations, this is of critical importance to the couple, such as the case of an Indian couple who wanted to make sure that their AID baby did not look like the child of a lower caste.

In one survey of AID couples, 40 percent had been told by friends and relatives that the child resembled the husband. One doctor reported the happy coincidence of a AID baby born with a kinked little finger on his left hand; the husband had the same finger kink, as did all the males in the husband's family.

· *FROZEN SPERM*

In recent years the infertility specialists have had an alternative to asking a medical student donor to step into the office and leave a sperm specimen about a half hour before the woman is due to be inseminated. Commercial sperm banks have sprung up in the past decade, allowing doctors to obtain frozen sperm from a faraway anonymous donor and defrost it before the insemination. According to the American Association of Tissue Banks, there are sixteen major sperm banks (known as cryobanks) in the United States.

The first suggestion for a bank of frozen sperm was made in 1866 by an Italian scientist as a means to save the sperm of a man going off to war and enable his wife to give birth to a legitimate child of the marriage even if her husband died on the battlefield. During the Vietnam War, the frozen sperm of some American soldiers was sent back to their wives in California so that they would be fathers by the time they returned home.

In 1953, three American babies were born who had been conceived with sperm that had been frozen. Since then, the use of frozen sperm has solved some of the problems inherent in the use of fresh sperm, but has given rise to its own difficulties. Fresh sperm retains its fertilizing ability for only about a half hour, a period too short to obtain reliable test results on the sperm or the donor before the insemination takes place. With frozen sperm, more extensive tests can be performed and the sperm can even be "quarantined" (as is bull sperm) for a month or so to see if the donor shows signs of an infection or other problem that was not recognized at the time of the donation.

The use of frozen sperm also permits a greater choice of donors. Physicians are not limited to donors in their geographical area; they can order sperm from a bank such as Idant in New York City, which maintains samples from about one hundred different donors. Sperm banks in Australia exchange semen in order to avoid the possibilty of an incestuous marriage between AID children from the same donor living in a small geographical area. "In Adelaide we use a donor for two pregnancies and then he [that is, his sperm] gets flown off to Melbourne," says an Australian doctor.

Curie-Cohen and his colleagues found that of those AID practitioners using primarily fresh sperm, only 8 percent were able to obtain donors from outside their geographical area. Of those using frozen, 68.1 percent used donors from outside their locality.

Certain men can be recruited as donors for a sperm bank who would not donate fresh sperm because their schedules do not allow them to be "on call" whenever a doctor has in his or her office a woman who is about to ovulate. Robert Klark Graham added a new twist to sperm banking when he solicited donations from Nobel Prize winners; he visited potential donors with the freezing equipment so that they would not even have to take the time to travel to his Escondido, California, bank.

Frozen sperm can be shipped anywhere. One New York fertility practitioner has shipped sperm to Honduras. The couple's initial chances of conception were thwarted, however, when customs officials opened the package and accidentally damaged the sperm.

Since a single donation is frozen into several separate straws for multiple inseminations, a couple who have one AID child can reserve straws from the same donor to create a second child in the future. Some couples report that they feel like a closer family when the same donor is used and the children thus resemble each other.

There are those who urge caution in the use of frozen sperm, though. "Uncertainties regarding the long-term genetic adequacy and biologic potency of frozen sperm, insufficient understanding of the relationship between cryopreservation and the fertilizing capability of sperm, and the absence of carefully controlled human studies of the safety and efficacy of various cryopreservation techniques now in use all suggest that semen cryobanking should be defined as an experimental procedure," wrote Mark Frankel in *Legal Medical Quarterly*. In 1972, a task force of the American Public Health Association and Planned Parenthood-World Population speculated that prolonged frozen storage of sperm could lead to genetic damage and birth defects. Speculation that the current freezing system will do genetic damage to the sperm does not seem to have been borne out, however. A report of five thousand children around the world who had been conceived with frozen sperm indicated that they were just as healthy as children conceived naturally.

More research is needed, however, on how long frozen sperm retains its ability to fertilize. Many experts suggest that sperm should be used within three years of its initial freezing, although children have been conceived through sperm frozen for up to twelve years.

Currently, the major problem with frozen sperm is that its success rate at achieving pregnancies is about 25 percent less than that of fresh sperm. Some studies show that sperm lose about 10 percent to 30 percent of their motility in the freezing and thawing process; the American Fertility Society speculates that the loss is closer to 50 percent. Thus, unless doctors freeze sperm that is superior to the type they use fresh, the chance of pregnancy is lessened.

Frozen sperm also has a shorter life span in a woman's reproductive tract than does fresh sperm. While fresh sperm will live for forty-eight hours, their frozen counterparts will last only about twenty-four hours. Doctors who use frozen sperm therefore must pinpoint a woman's time of ovulation more accurately than do doctors using fresh sperm, so that both egg and sperm will be alive and ready to mate at the same time. As increasingly sophisticated methods of pinpointing ovulation come into more widespread use (such as blood tests measuring hormones or ultrasound measurements of ovarian follical size), the pregnancy rate with frozen sperm will undoubtedly rise.

In France, where frozen semen is widely used, the success rates are fairly high. A study of 2,193 French women undergoing AID with sperm that had been frozen found that within a year of attempts, 73 percent of the women under age twenty-five conceived, as did 74.1 percent of the twenty-five-to-thirty age group, 61.5 percent of the thirty-one-to-thirty-five age group, and 53.6 percent of the women over age thirty-five. Right now, frozen sperm is used for only 13 percent of all inseminations in the United States. But because frozen sperm allows more screening and a wider range of donors, it may become the first choice approach of most AID specialists in the next decade.

• *THE PROCESS OF ARTIFICIAL INSEMINATION*

If you and your husband decide to use AID, you will need to keep a basal body temperature chart and discuss it with your doctor so that he or she can perform the insemination around the time of ovulation. The physician should also check your cervical mucus and the dilation of your cervix and inseminate only if the cervix is "ripe."

The doctor will inseminate you on what appears to be the day before you ovulate. If your temperature does not rise the next morning (indicating ovulation has occurred), he or she will ask you to return for a second insemination two days after the first attempt in case the egg was released later than expected.

Some couples are afraid to ask questions about what artificial insemination entails and consequently are frightened by the thought of the procedure. Some women worry that it will require surgery. Others think they will have to have intercourse with the donor.

The insemination procedure is not at all complex. "With all of the thinking, counseling, evaluation, and planning that must proceed AID, the actual insemination process is so simple that is is almost anticlimactic," wrote Dr. William W. Beck, Jr., in the journal *Fertility and Sterility*. You will be asked to lie down in the position used for a routine pelvic exam. A vaginal speculum will be inserted and semen will then either be squirted directly into the vagina against the cervix or put into a cap like a diaphragm that is placed on the cervix. A minority of doctors inject the semen directly into the uterus, but most advise against such action. The benefits obtained by proximity to the egg are outweighted by increased likelihood of causing an infection. Also, insertion of more than one half cubic centimeter of sperm into the uterus may cause cramping and the uterus may contract, expelling the sperm. In contrast, when sperm is deposited by cap or injection near the cervix, the process is entirely painless. After an insemination in which sperm is injected, you will remain lying on your back for up to thirty minutes so the sperm will have an opportunity to travel to your fallopian tubes. If the cap method is used, you can get up after ten minutes and keep the cap in place for four to six hours.

The process of insemination is so simple that a number of couples, as well as some single women, have accomplished do-it-yourself inseminations using a drugstore syringe or a turkey baster. A home insemination kit is even in the works for possible marketing to infertile couples, who presumably would then be able to buy semen directly from sperm banks.

• *SHOULD YOU MIX SPERM?*

Some doctors offer couples the option of having the oligospermic husband's sperm mixed with that of the donor. They do so to provide a psychological benefit to the husband, who can then believe that it was *his* sperm that created the child. One California infertility specialist reports that, when given the choice, 75 percent of the husbands he treats choose to have their sperm mixed with that of the donor.

Recent research, however, warns against mixing sperm since the addition of the husband's sperm can reduce the fertilizating power of that of the donor. Instead, practitioners suggest that the husband and wife make love on the night of the insemination after the donor sperm have had their initial opportunity at fertilization.

• *HOW LONG SHOULD YOU KEEP TRYING?*

The success rate of individual doctors in achieving pregnancies through AID varies greatly. Recent reports in medical journals reported an average AID treatment length before pregnancy that ranged from 2.5 months to 9.5 months.

A study done at the Tyler Medical Clinic at the University of California at Los Angeles found that a substantial percentage of couples dropped out after a few attempts at AID. A similar study at Baylor University in Houston reported a 21 percent dropout rate after only two cycles.

"Infertile couples tend to blame themselves or see themselves as failures," observes AID counselor Betty Orlandino. "Although it takes an average of three to six months of insemination for conception to occur using artificial insemination, an infertile couple will often drop out after the first unsuccessful insemination."

It is almost as if the couple were thinking, "If we don't get pregnant in the first or second month, it wasn't meant to happen." They seem to forget that AID does not promise immediate success; even fertile couples have only a 20 percent chance per month of achieving a pregnancy through normal intercourse.

Still, it is not wise to continue indefinitely with AID. Yes, pregnancies have occurred after three years of treatment, but you should probably reassess after six months and consider whether something new should be tried to enhance your chances of an AID pregnancy.

Although painless, extended treatment with AID has many disadvantages; costs mount and it is terribly distracting to have to drop everything once or twice a month to see a physician for inseminations. One doctor found that of 605 couples seeking AID from him, over a third (277) gave up for financial reasons or because the wife decided she did not like the procedure.

After six months of trying to achieve an AID pregnancy, approach your doctor with questions about improving your chances. Often, poor timing of the insemination is at fault and a more accurate means of pinpointing ovulation is necessary. Ask your doctor whether he or she will consider using blood tests to gauge your time of ovulation or whether an expert radiologist can read an ultrasound scan closely enough to predict when one of your ovarian follicles will rupture and release an egg. Or you might ask about the possibility of using clomiphene citrate to regulate your ovulation so that the doctor is not wasting inseminations in months when you have not released an egg at all. If your doctor does not offer these options, consider finding someone else who does. Curie-Cohen and his colleagues found that some doctors had a 20 percent success rate with AID, while others had a 100 percent success rate. Doctors with large practices tended to have higher success rates.

• *THE EMOTIONAL ASPECTS OF AID*

Although the physical process of artificial insemination is well understood, the emotional effects of the procedure have been neglected. In 1963, psychiatrist Gerda Gerstel published an article stating that "a decision to participate in artificial donor insemination, in itself, is indicative of an emotional disturbance." This insensitive notion was based on Gerstel's therapy with a small group of couples in which the wives had undergone AID. These five couples had come to Gerstel precisely because they were upset about the husband's infertility and the AID process. Gerstel's analysis overlooked the thousands of other couples who had no psychological problems after becoming parents via AID.

The emotional side of AID does not consist of a lone reaction. Rather, participants describe a series of intense feelings that occur at various points in the process. All should be understood and deftly dealt with as the need arises.

Many men are traumatized by the knowledge that they are infertile and unlikely to father a child biologically. Too often, though, that assault to the emotions is followed immediately by the suggestion that they allow their wife to conceive by another man through AID. Men need time to deal with the knowledge of their infertility before confronting a radical method for dealing with it.

"I really take the medical profession to task for saying 'We've just learned that we can't do anything about Joe's sperm, but we'll get you a donor. Let's see, Beth, you're ovulating in ten days, why don't we start then?'" complains psychologist Aphrodite Clamar. "There needs to be a mourning period after the man learns of his infertility, but few doctors let it happen."

"The doctor says to the man, 'Nobody will know about your infertility, she'll be pregnant, it will be your kid, it will all be fine,'" protests Los Angeles psychotherapist Annette Baran. "There is no explanation of the feelings. It is just all frosted over."

It is crucial for the husband to be able to talk out his feelings with his wife or a counselor or in a support group before his wife agrees to be inseminated. Some men quickly agree to AID because they want to save face and feel that adopting a child will force them to admit their infertility to family and friends. "Or a man may plunge into AID, even though he may be ambivalent or secretly opposed because he feels he has no right to stand in the way of his wife's biological right to have a child," notes Richard Amelar.

"The husband may agree to AID because he doesn't want to feel he has put his wife in the position of choosing between him and a baby," Clamar comments.

If any of these rationales is behind your agreement to AID, you should postpone the AID decision until you have given it more thought. Counseling may even be necessary to help you both determine whether you will be comfortable with the AID decision.

Thoughtful conversations between you and your spouse are also necessary to clear up any concerns either of you have about the donor. Some husbands feel that AID is akin to letting a wife sleep with another man. It may be necessary for the wife to emphasize the scientific nature of the process and assure her husband of her love for him. "He needs to realize that 'being a father' means rearing a child, not contributing genetic materials to his conception," writes Dr. Donald Goldstein of Harvard Medical School.

Carol and Jim Jordan (not their real names) were two months into an AID pregnancy when Jim realized that things had moved too quickly for him. He told Carol he had had a change of heart and insisted that she have an abortion. She did. Four years later, though, Jim had come to terms with his infertility and he and Carol were able to initiate AID with both sharing the excitement of the impending pregnancy.

Wives have their own psychological reactions to AID. They sometimes feel selfish that their genetic heritage will live on, while their husband's will not. They often remark, "I wanted to have *his* baby," and point to cherished mental and physical characteristics of their husbands that will be lost to future generations.

If the AID process is hurried without sufficient explanation or if the woman senses that her husband is ambivalent or distant, her emotional reaction may translate into anovulation, causing the attempted insemination to fail.

"The couple needs time to mourn and grieve for the child they will never have, their biological child," advises Baran. "They need time to explore their feelings. Otherwise, there may be problems later on. The husband may feel like a fraud when congratulated on the birth of the child. The power structure may change in the family so that the woman may feel it is really her baby and the man may be unable to discipline and set limits on the child."

"It's better to get these negative feelings out sooner than later," Baran continues. "Many times these negatives can be turned into positives by openly confronting them in the light of day."

The importance of an open discussion of feelings is illustrated in a case handled by Amelar. On a joint visit, the couple had told him they did not want to undergo AID. When Amelar saw the wife alone, however, she asked if she could be inseminated with donor semen with the husband thinking it was his. In another private conversation the husband said he thought that the wife would not be willing to undergo AID, but asked if she could be inseminated with donor sperm and told it was the husband's.

"Of course, the answer to both was no," states Amelar, "but it's a starting point to get the couple to think about it together."

In her research on AID couples, Baran has found that when couples seek AID for genetic reasons or because the husband underwent a vasectomy after having children in a previous marriage, they experience less psychological trauma than do infertile couples who choose AID. In the former instances, the husband does not feel his virility is threatened and the couple feels that they are entering into AID as a matter of choice, rather than having it forced upon them.

In 1976, Dr. Amnon David and Dalia Avidan published an in-depth psychological study of forty-four AID couples. By using a questionnaire and psychologists' interviews with the couples, the researchers learned that 80 percent of the infertile husbands had guilt feelings. They felt unable to fulfill the expectation of society—and their wives—that they would become fathers. Ironically, the wives also felt guilty; they were caught in a conflict between sharing their husbands' failure and reveling in their pregnancy.

Much of the guilt associated with AID comes from the exclusion of the husbands from the process. The wife feels awkward that she is getting pregnant without her husband. The husband has thoughts that he has let his wife down and is contributing nothing to the pregnancy.

"The husband may feel, 'This is her baby. I didn't contribute. All I'm doing is paying the bill,'" says Clamar.

Guilt feelings can be cleared up by encouraging husbands to attend the clinic with their wives. Some doctors involve husbands even more actively in the process.

"The more enlightened doctors are letting the husband do the insemination, just as obstetricians are now involving husbands in the delivery," Clamar points out. "This helps integrate the husband, so they begin as a family unit."

Some doctors put the husband in charge of keeping track of the basal body temperature and bringing the wife in when she is about to ovulate. In the clinic, they allow the husband to insert the syringe and introduce the sperm into the woman's vagina and then the couple shares the half hour wait, keeping their fingers crossed that a pregnancy will occur. Some physicians even teach the husband to do the inseminations at home.

The emotional spectrum does not end once insemination begins, however. "Some men experience temporary potency problems, and both may experience loss of libido at this time," writes Barbara Menning in "Psycho-Social Issues in Donor Insemination." "I encourage couples to communicate as honestly as possible with each other, to 'confess' their fears and to share physical comfort simply in holding each other until a mutual sexual response returns—usually very quickly."

Couples may also be fearful that their AID child will be born with a defect or that the child will be radically different from them in appearance. "These fears most often surface right after news of a successful conception," writes Menning, and "often peak again right before the time of delivery."

According to Menning, such fears are more accentuated than the fertile pregnant couple's concern about their biological child, but are still understandable. "The couple quite literally place 'blind faith' in the hands of the physician and his or her staff, and it is logical that they might have rational and irrational fears over a 'mistake,'" notes Menning. If couples insist on more communication with the doctor about selection of the donor, such fears should be lessened.

If both the husband and wife have been open about their feelings about AID and come to terms with their emotions, the pregnancy can be a stunningly happy time for them. The satisfaction that most couples ultimately feel about the baby born to them through AID is reflected by their willingness to undergo the process again. Ninety-eight percent of those couples who bear a child via AID feel their decision was the right one and a majority of those who have AID children decide to have another child in the same manner.

Early opponents of AID worried that the procedure would drive a wedge into the marriage. They believed that the biological relationship of the child to only one parent (as opposed to both or neither) would cause extreme tension and upset the delicate balance of the family structure. But AID marriages have proven to be stable ones. In fact, a couple with an AID child is more likely to stay married than is a couple with a natural child. AID couples have a divorce rate of around 1 percent, substantially lower than the overall divorce rate of 49.6 percent. In many ways, the strength of their marriage has already been tested by their reaction to infertility and the soul-searching decision-making process that led to artificial insemination. The couple usually comes to AID assured of their love for each other, and the birth of an AID child that is a product of that love brings them even closer together. According to the American Fertility Society, "in most cases, it [AID] has strengthened the bonds of marriage of those participating, rather than weakening them."

• *SOCIETY'S REACTION TO AID*

While AID seems to knit a couple together, they wonder about how those around them will take the news. Seven years after the birth of their AID child, one couple finally told the husband's mother about the husband's infertility and their use of donor semen to conceive. She appeared to accept the news well, but cautioned her son, "Don't tell your father. He may not love his grandchild as much if he knows."

Some of the negative social reaction to AID is due to a misunderstanding about the process. If you decide to tell friends or relatives about your use of AID, you may need to reassure them that it does not involve intercourse with a stranger and that there is absolutely nothing artificial about the pregnancy once it is under way.

Beyond family and friends, though, a larger societal opposition to AID focuses on the concern that the procedure will be used in a demeaning way to breed people like animals or to create individuals for particular societal roles as in *Brave New World.* Julian Huxley, in *The Uniqueness of Man,* pointed the way for that possibility by suggesting that artificial insemination by donor "opened up new horizons . . . to man and woman to consummate the sexual function with those whom on perhaps quite other grounds they admire."

Already there has been a run on a British sperm bank thought to have Mick Jagger's sperm, and apparently Robert Klark Graham has attracted couples who want to have artificial insemination with the sperm of a Nobel Prize winner. The publicity surrounding these isolated incidents clouds the fact that most couples are not trying to create a superchild, but rather are trying to "adopt" sperm from a healthy male whose characteristics resemble that of the husband.

• *RELIGIOUS CONSIDERATIONS ABOUT AID*

The couple's decision to undertake AID, as well as their feeling about disclosing that decision, may be shaped by religious considerations as well. The Catholic church has staunchly opposed AID ever since Pope Pius XII spoke out against it in 1949. Pope Pius XII rejected the procedure on the basis of the encyclical of Pope Pius XI, which stated that the exclusive right of procreation remained within marriage.

"Artificial insemination in marriage, but produced by the active element of a third person is . . . immoral, and, as such, to be condemned outright," declared Pope Pius XII in 1949. "The husband and wife alone have the reciprocal right over their bodies in order to engender a new life; and this right is exclusive, untransferable, inalienable."

The Pope had other concerns: he felt AID placed people on the level of beasts and exposed society to grave danger. In addition, he felt, "to reduce cohabitation of married persons and the conjugal act to a mere organic function for the germ of life would be to convert the domestic hearth and sanctuary of the family into nothing more than a biological laboratory." Within the Catholic faith, AID is viewed as adultery and the child is illegitimate.

The Lutheran church, most Anglican churches, and the Orthodox Jewish faith also oppose AID. In some instances, though, Orthodox Jews have been granted consent by their rabbis to undergo the procedure. "Among the very Orthodox Jews, the rabbis who have consented insist that the donor not be Jewish," notes Amelar. "They want to assure that a half-brother and half-sister do not unwittingly marry each other."

Within the Protestant church and Reform Judaism, the procedure is viewed with less hostility. In fact, at least one Reform Jewish rabbi has become an AID father.

• *LEGAL ISSUES INVOLVING AID*

When *in vitro* fertilization is used, the genetic parents are the couple rearing the child. That is not true with AID, where a sperm donor enters the picture, raising legal issues about the rights and responsibilities of the donor and the infertile husband.

In AID, those issues have been litigated in the courts, usually after one of those rare breakups of the marriage of a couple who have an AID child. In the divorce action, former husbands have alleged that they should not have to support the AID child, since they are not genetically related. The women have sometimes asked that their former husbands not be allowed to see the child based on that same rationale. Before no-fault divorce, some men who wished to obtain a divorce alleged that wives who had undergone AID were guilty of adultery.

The cases involving AID have resulted in varied outcomes. A 1954 Illinois case held that an AID is adulterous, even when the husband consents. In an early Canadian AID case, the judge applied similar logic and held that adultery did not require having intercourse with another. That judge defined adultery as the voluntary surrender of one's reproductive powers, which he felt a woman did when undergoing AID.

The more recent (and better) approach is typified by a California judge who notes the absurdity of the viewpoint that the AID recipient commits adultery with the doctor or donor. The judge wrote, "Since the doctor may be a woman, or the husband himself may administer the insemination by a syringe, this is patently absurd; to consider it an act of adultery with the donor, who at the time of insemination may be a thousand miles away or may even be dead, is equally absurd."

Similarly, a New York judge has written: "An AID child is not 'begotten' by a father who is not the husband; the donor is anonymous; the wife does not have sexual intercourse or commit adultery with him; if there is any 'begetting' it is by the doctor, who in this specialty is often a woman. The suggestion that the husband might not regard the child as his own has been dispelled by our gratifying experience with adoptive parents. Since there is consent by the husband, there is no marital infidelity."

As to the status of the child, a 1963 New York court held an AID child to be illegitimate. However, even in cases such as that, where the courts have not viewed AID children as legitimate, the judges have protected the child, relying upon the husband's consent to the AID process to hold him liable for support for the child. A subsequent New York case, a decade later, held that the infertile father was indeed the legal father. The court stated: "It serves no purpose whatsoever to stigmatize the AID child; or to compel the parent formally to adopt in order to confer upon the AID child the status and rights of a naturally conceived child."

Even in cases where the AID child was not held to be the legitimate child of the husband, the donor has never involuntarily been required to support the child. "The anonymous donor of the sperm cannot be considered the 'natural father,' as he is no more responsible for the use made of his sperm than is the donor of blood or a kidney," wrote the judge in the California AID case.

In a recent New Jersey case, however, the donor sued to win visitation rights to the child. This was a most unusual case, though, since the donor knew the woman who had used his sperm. In fact, at the time, he and the woman were dating. She refused to have pre-marital sex but did want a premarital pregnancy, so they visited a sperm bank to inquire about using its facilities. The doctor at the sperm bank turned them away, but, in the course of the conversation, provided them with enough information to do the artificial insemination themselves. Three months into the pregnancy, though, the woman severed her relationship with the donor. He sued to be able to see the child. In these unusual circumstances, the court granted the donor visitation rights, although he was required to furnish child support as a prerequisite to such rights. This case provides no precedent, however, for an anonymous donor to sue for visitation rights to the child you have conceived with his sperm.

So far, none of the court cases discussing AID has dealt with the inheritance rights of the child. This may be because most AID children have not yet reached an age where their social fathers have died. After all, widespread use of AID did not begin until the past few decades, so there are relatively few AID-conceived individuals who are over the age of thirty-five and probably few fathers over the age of seventy-five.

Precautions should be taken to help ensure that your AID child is viewed as the legitimate offspring of your marriage. You and your spouse should prepare a written consent that is witnessed by someone, such as your doctor. You should also prepare wills that specifically grant rights to your AID child by name. If John Doe just states in his will that he leaves money and property to his son (intending it to refer to John, Jr., the child born to his wife through AID), relatives might challenge the will claiming John, Jr. should get nothing because he isn't really a son.

Already, in Scandinavia, relatives have successfully claimed that the child of a couple was not their legitimate child and thus should have no right to inherit. After the husband's death, the relatives proved to the court that he had been sterile and therefore the child was not his child. The court granted the child no money at all. Although it is hard to predict whether American courts would be that harsh, you can avoid the possibility by referring to an AID child by the full name—for example, John Doe, Jr.

• *AID LAWS*

Because of the confusion in the AID cases, nearly half the states have adopted laws to cover AID. When the issue initially came before state lawmakers, it was too emotionally charged for rational consideration to prevail. A man who sponsored three pro-AID bills in the Minnesota legislature said he was subject to "unbelievable personal abuse" and received "vicious, anonymous calls by the hundreds."

In the 1950s, a bill was proposed in the Ohio legislature that would fine everyone involved with AID $500 and subject them to one to five years in prison. The couple, the donor, and even the physician would have been criminals under the proposed law.

Luckily, the law never passed, and the laws that were adopted, starting in the mid-1960s, all favor AID. Now twenty-four states have AID laws, although they vary widely in their approach and no law addresses all the legal issues that AID could entail.

Most of the twenty-four state laws follow the pattern that if a married woman is artificially inseminated with the consent of her husband, the child is the legal child of that couple. The statutes vary in the additional requirements they make. Fourteen require that a physician or someone under a physician's supervision perform the procedure. Eleven require that artificial insemination records be filed with a state agency, but indicate that such records are confidential and can only be inspected pursuant to a court order. All statutes require the husband's consent and most (nineteen states) require the consent be in writing. Only the Oregon statute specifically addresses the issue of artificial insemination of a single woman: it holds that AID may be performed on any woman with her written consent.

Eleven states expressly sever the legal connection between the donor and child by providing, in general, that a donor is *not* the father of the child if he provides semen to a woman other than his wife. If such a law had been in effect in New Jersey, presumably the man who donated sperm for the artificial insemination of the woman he was dating would probably have had no liability for support even though he was a known rather than an anonymous donor.

The statutes provide very little guidance about how donors should be selected. The city of New York has regulated the selection of AID donors since 1949, providing that carriers of genetic diseases or defects and men suffering from venereal disease or tuberculosis cannot be donors. The ordinance also provides that the donor and recipient must have compatible Rh factors. On the state level, only the Oregon statute provides screening guidelines—that a *doctor* must select the donor and that the donor must be free from any genetic or venereal disease.

Only the Georgia law addresses the liability of the doctor. It says that doctors who perform artificial insemination with the consent of a husband and wife shall be relieved of civil liability to the couple of the child for the results, except that doctors are liable for negligent administration or performance of AID.

According to attorney Sharon Steeves, new laws should be passed to ensure the genetic integrity of sperm. For example, she contends that "local governments should undertake increased control over sperm banks and genetic screening of potential donors."

As you can see, the court decisions and the statutes do not provide all the answers about how doctors should conduct an AID practice. They do not discuss legal liabilities in the rare situation that the child is born with a genetic defect, nor do they address whether an AID child may win the right to see records about the genetic father, the sperm donor, nor do they generally deal with the accessibility of AID to couples who are *not* married or single women who wish an AID child.

With proper donor screening there is very little risk that an AID child will be born with a genetic defect. However, as in the case of a natural pregnancy, that risk cannot be entirely eliminated. If the child does have a defect that could not have been anticipated or avoided through careful medical practice, there is no legal liability on the part of the doctor.

Doctors are certainly not required to provide a warranty that every AID child is free of genetic defects. Rather, their responsibilities with respect to an AID pregnancy are much the same as with *any* pregnancy—they must advise the couple about screening for common genetic disorders and about amniocentesis. If a doctor is negligent in these respects and the child is born with a serious defect, the couple (and perhaps the child, too) would have a right to sue the doctor. Some doctors have couples sign a form that says that the doctor is not liable if the woman gets an infection from the insemination or the child is born with a defect as a result of the doctor's negligence. A court would probably *still* let a couple sue, even if they had signed such an agreement, if the doctor were clearly negligent. Courts have held that doctors cannot excuse themselves from liability for negligence merely by having a patient sign a form to that effect.

• *AID AND THE SINGLE WOMAN*

There is yet another legal area concerning AID that deserves mention. In some instances, unmarried women want to undergo AID. They may be single and living alone, or be living with an infertile man in a long-standing loving relationship, or they may be involved in a lesbian relationship.

I have received a number of calls from doctors saying they have an unmarried woman patient who wants to become pregnant through AID. They usually say the woman is well-adjusted, has received glowing ratings from a psychologist, and would be a good mother. They ask me for legal advice about what they should do. Some of these doctors seem afraid that if they do AID for a single woman, the courts will start looking for a "father" for the child and slap the doctor with a paternity suit. I think this is a far-fetched, unrealistic fear.

Although states other than Oregon do not legally sanction AID for a single woman, there are certainly no laws that *forbid* it. Of course, doctors who are in private practice, not affiliated with a state university, can turn down patients for virtually any reason they wish. If you are an unmarried woman seeking AID from a private practitioner, be sure to tell him or her that the process is not illegal and that he or she need not be fearful of liability for treating you. Also point out that a national survey of AID practitioners found that one in ten does artificial insemination of single women. The Sperm Bank of Northern California caters to single women, and at the Southern California Cryobank in Los Angeles, 15 percent of the customers are single women.

If you are an unmarried woman, your legal right to AID is greatest if you consult a practitioner at a clinic that is affiliated with a state university. He or she may not turn you away so readily. The U.S. Supreme Court has held that the constitutional rights to privacy protects the procreation decisions of both married and single people. The government, whether through a law or the action of the employee of a state or city university, cannot interfere with that right except in a narrow way to further a compelling interest. Think about the arguments a clinic might make to justify excluding single women. They might claim that they want to ensure for the child a psychologically and financially sound home. A court would probably *not* be willing to uphold a ban on a single woman on those grounds, however, since obviously there are some well-off, well-balanced unmarried women who would make good parents.

There has already been one case on the subject. A thirty-six-year-old woman sued Wayne State University's AID clinic because it restricted AID to married couples. With the American Civil Liberties Union representing her, she alleged that the clinic's policy violated her right to privacy and to equal protection. She said in her affidavit that although she was interested in remarrying, she felt she must bear a child in the next year or so because of her age. She pointed out that whether she remarried or not, she felt competent to be a parent and provide for all of her child's emotional, financial, and social needs. The case never got to court, though; it was settled with the university's agreement to drop its marriage requirement and to consider the woman for its AID program.

"The key point is that each woman has a right to decide by herself whether to procreate," explains Philadelphia attorney Barbara Kritchevsky. "Absent a compelling interest, outsiders may not constitutionally legislate their beliefs about the desirability of any adult woman bearing a child."

Single women have already won the right to be parents in other areas of law. All states allow unmarried people to adopt. Various cases have granted lesbians custody of children. In one case, the court granted custody to the deceased mother's lesbian lover instead of to the child's married aunt. Although the psychological effect on the child is always the most important concern, judges are beginning to put aside their stereotypes and consider the individual situation. In response to the argument that children in the custody of a lesbian mother would be emotionally harmed by community intolerance, one judge wrote, "It is just as reasonable to expect that they will emerge better equipped to search out their own standards of right and wrong, better able to perceive that the majority is not always correct in its moral judgments, and better able to understand the importance of conforming their beliefs to the requirements of reason and tested knowledge, not the constraints of currently popular sentiment or prejudice."

The use of AID by single women may provide a benefit for couples. By and large, single women communicate openly about their choice of AID— and tell their children. This may help society become more adjusted to the notion of artificial insemination in general and could lead to greater communication and support among those children who are told by their parents of their special origins.

• *POSTHUMOUS AID*

As AID is used more frequently and in more unique ways the legal issues become more complicated. Already, New Jersey attorney

Winthrop D. Thies, writing in the journal *Trusts and Estates,* has suggested that there ought to be a law to protect the financial interests of AID children who are conceived *after* the father's death.

This science fiction-sounding scenario has already occurred. Roberto Casali learned that he had cancer. Before starting chemotherapy, he had some of his sperm frozen as "fertility insurance." After his death, his wife, Kim, was inseminated with his sperm and gave birth to their third child.

Another couple, both professional athletes, delayed marriage. When they finally got married, they learned that he had pancreatic cancer. They stored his semen so that she could get pregnant while he was being treated for cancer. She was successfully inseminated, but he died before the child was born. She later had a second child by him, conceived by artificial insemination after his death.

"We have a number of men who have provided for the use of their sperm after their death," says Roxanne Feldschuh, director of the Idant sperm bank in New York. Idant will continue storing sperm and allow the wife to be inseminated after her husband dies if the man has designated it in his will. Yet questions may still arise regarding who owns that frozen sperm. Could, for example, the wife donate it to be used by someone else for AID? If her husband were famous, could she sell the sperm to women who were his fans?

• *THE FUTURE OF AID*

Asked "What do you think of sex?", Marilyn Monroe replied, "I think sex is here to stay!" Relying on that quote, British attorney Lord Kilbrandon has stated, "I think AID is here to stay. . . . [T]he law has got to consider AID not in a prohibitory way and perhaps only in a regulatory way so far as is required to make the technique acceptable to society."

8 ❦ Surrogate Mothers

Jane and Marc Kloner have been married for thirteen years. They have pursued various infertility treatments for the past nine years in order to bring a child into their lives. Jane even tried one attempt at *in vitro* fertilization. As it became clear that modern medicine could not readily offer them a baby, the Kloners began to think about exploring other possibilities, from adoption to remaining childless.

"Sometimes when you want something so much, you lose sight of what it is you really want," confesses Jane. "I've really had to stand back and ask do I really want children or do I just want to solve this problem."

The answer to Jane's question came in the form of a month-long visit from a seven-year-old and a four-year-old, the children of one of her friends. "I realized that children would fit in well," Jane recalls. "My husband and I have been devoting all of our life to just the two of us. It would be great to share with children."

Jane was ready to try adoption, but Marc felt that if there was any way possible to have a biologically connected child, he would like that. They decided they would seek a surrogate mother.

A surrogate mother is a woman who is inseminated with the sperm of a man whose own wife is not capable of conceiving or carrying a child to term. She carries the child for the nine months and then, after its birth, allows the couple to adopt the baby. "I think of myself as a human incubator," says Elizabeth Kane, a Pekin, Illinois, woman who, for a fee, served as a surrogate for a childless couple.

• *WHO SHOULD USE A SURROGATE MOTHER?*

The surrogate mother is a viable alternative whether the cause of a woman's infertility is a malfunction that prevents her ovaries from producing eggs, a malady that has damaged her tubes, or a hysterectomy. A woman who is fearful of passing on a serious genetic defect might also wish to use a surrogate, as would a woman who has been advised by her doctor not to get pregnant because of high blood pressure, diabetes, or other physical problems. Surrogate mothering has an advantage over adoption of requiring only a nine-month or so wait and producing a child that is genetically the child of the husband. Also, unlike adoption, the couple has some choice over the type of woman who will be carrying their child.

Since producing a child through a surrogate mother does not require any biological input from the infertile wife, it is available when other treatments are scarce or when no other option is available. For example, while embryo transfer could be used on a woman whose ovaries or tubes are not functioning, this technique is being offered in only a few centers across the country. Surrogate mothering, however, is potentially widely available. In some situations, such as when a woman's uterus and ovaries have been removed or damaged, surrogate mothering offers the only hope of procreation of a child genetically related to the couple.

• *WHEN SHOULD YOU USE A SURROGATE MOTHER?*

While artificial insemination has been widely available for at least forty years to women whose husbands are infertile, very little has been available to help women who themselves were completely sterile. This has been a particular irony since women, more so than men, are emotionally devastated when they find out they are infertile. After all, it is the woman in our culture who has been raised to be a mother from the time she fed and changed the diapers on her first doll. It is the woman who has the main responsibility for birth control and who may feel like a fool when she discovers at age twenty-seven or thirty-two or thirty-five that she is sterile after all those years of fumbling with a diaphragm or risking the side effects of the Pill and maybe even panicking over a slightly late period, thinking it was an unwanted pregnancy.

Now, though, a surrogate mother offers hope for all couples who cannot bear their own child because of female infertility. Yet not all couples who *could* use a surrogate *should*. There may be an alternative solution to their infertility problem that would allow them to bear their own child; even if there is not, surrogate parenthood may be inadvisable as too emotionally risky for them.

If you are considering using a surrogate, go back and read Chapter Three to make sure that you have not overlooked a treatment that could provide a medical solution to your infertility problem. One drawback with most surrogate programs is that they make no independent check of the wife's reproductive system. Thus, couples may be seeking surrogates even when there is a chance they could conceive naturally. (In the *in vitro* programs, the women are examined again even if previous doctors have said they were infertile. In many cases, the couples who thought they would need to undergo the test-tube baby technique learn that they could conceive naturally with some other treatment.)

If you have tubal problems and are considering hiring a surrogate, you may want to give some thought to using *in vitro* fertilization (IVF) instead. In addition to allowing you to conceive a child that is genetically related to both you and your spouse, if IVF is successful in one of its initial attempts, it will be less expensive than hiring a surrogate.

If you and your spouse decide that, physically, surrogate parenthood is the best solution to your infertility problem, the two of you will still need to spend considerable time discussing whether you will be able to handle the emotional complexities of the process. You must have not only accepted your own infertility but also analyzed how you will resolve your feelings about the surrogate.

The use of a stand-in childbearer (who donates the egg and womb) is naturally more emotionally troublesome to a woman than is the use of artificial insemination by a donor. With AID, once the couple has made the decision to have the treatment, the pregnancy proceeds quite normally for the woman. A child, her child, is growing inside her. Moreover, the woman, the person with the genetic tie to the child born of artificial insemination, is the parent who ultimately spends the most time with the child.

Since the prime child-rearing responsibilities will almost always be the woman's, she must explore her feelings deeply before she and her husband decide to invite a surrogate mother to bear a child for them. The main question she must ask herself is, Will I feel this child is "our" child?

Her husband must also explore his reasons for wanting a surrogate. One New York man wanted to have a child via a surrogate to hold his shaky marriage together. The surrogate became pregnant, but the man and his wife separated before the child was born.

Another man contacted the Association for Surrogate Parenting Services, Inc., in Columbus, Ohio, asking for a surrogate who was an accomplished cellist. He would not accept a woman who merely appreciated music or played another sort of musical instrument.

"Anyone who sets up those kind of barriers cannot be serious about the process," says Kathryn Wyckoff, director of the program. She advises people who voice hard-to-meet requirements to reevaluate their commitment to surrogate motherhood.

Gene and Lynn (not their real names) are considering using a surrogate. Lynn feels that adopting a child would be preferable since it would put both her and her husband in an equal biological relationship with the child. But Gene will not even consider adoption. "I want a son that will be *mine*," he insists. Despite her misgivings, she is about to agree, in part because she feels "ashamed" that she has "failed as a wife to Gene" by not being able to give him his son.

Anyone spending a few minutes with Lynn will realize she is not ready yet for this major step. She acts guiltily, looks frazzled, and makes the nervous gestures of a person who feels she is facing an unsolvable problem. She needs to realize that rushing into parenting at this moment would not be fair to the child, who might not receive the full panoply of loving attention that Lynn is capable of.

It is also unfair to Lynn to pressure her in this way. Finding out six months earlier that she is sterile was unsettling enough. She now needs a cooling-off period to come to grips with that news before she can decide whether she can ever reach the point where she can think of a child carried by a surrogate as "her" child, too.

One method of determining whether you are ready to employ a surrogate is the jealousy test. How jealous are you that another woman will be carrying your husband's child? "It's natural to be jealous," advises Pennsylvania psychologist Howard Adelman, "but that should be overshadowed by the desire to have a child." You are ready for a surrogate if you can picture yourself in the place of infertile women like Donna, who said she got goosebumps when she heard her surrogate was pregnant, or Susan, who said about the baby her surrogate bore, "I feel as if I had carried him."

Surrogate mothering should not be rushed into. There is time to carefully consider whether it is right for you and, if it is, at what time. One advantage of surrogate mothering is that since the wife does not physically take part in the reproductive process, she does not have to speed the process for fear that her reproductive clock will run out. She does not have to hurry into childbearing like the woman who gets married in her mid-thirties and feels she must begin having children immediately before she goes into menopause. In fact, recent surveys show a growing number of relationships and marriages between older women and younger men—and these couples may become prime users of surrogates. In such a case, a woman who could no longer bear children herself could still see to it that her younger husband has a chance to have a child that is genetically his.

• *THE MEDICAL ASPECTS OF SURROGATE PARENTING*

The medical aspects of surrogate parenting begin, in some programs, with a thorough physical of the surrogate. In a Los Angeles surrogate program, infertility specialist Dr. William Karow undertakes an extensive workup on the surrogate. This can lead to some surprises. At least two potential surrogates who have come to his office were already pregnant by their own mates but did not realize it.

The programs vary in whether they require a physical of the

man who will be providing the sperm. Dr. Richard Levin's program in Louisville, Kentucky, requires the man to undergo a complete physical initially supplemented by tests for venereal disease each time he donates sperm.

Unlike the intricate procedure of egg removal and fertilization used in the test-tube baby technique and the painstaking process of flushing and implantation used in embryo adoption, the medical aspect of surrogate mothering is very simple. The process used is artificial insemination.

Initially, however, when couples began to request their doctors to aid in the insemination of a surrogate, the doctors refused. "When Sue volunteered to be a surrogate for George and Debbie, they couldn't find a doctor who was willing to help," recounts Dearborn, Michigan, attorney Noel Keane. "The doctors were all afraid they might be doing something illicit."

The threesome finally handled the matter themselves. Debbie purchased a diabetic syringe at the drug store and filled it with her husband's sperm. Following the directions in a family medical guide, she successfully injected the sperm into her friend Sue, a twenty-four-year-old virgin, and their child was born nine months later. Other couples have done inseminations with a turkey baster.

Now, however, there are a growing number of doctors who are sympathetic to the plight of couples who request insemination of a surrogate. In Levin's high-rise medical suite, the procedure is typical. The husband's semen is collected in one examining room while the surrogate mother waits to receive it in another. When artificial insemination is done as a medical procedure, the doctor involved can do a better job than the couple at estimating when the surrogate has ovulated, and time the insemination so that it takes place at a time when fertilization will be most likely.

The procedure takes place quickly. "It took more time for a television crew to set up their cameras to film an insemination than it did to perform it," observes Levin. The longest part of the process is the ten minutes to half hour after the insemination, during which the surrogate must rest quietly to give the sperm a chance to reach their appointed meeting place with her egg.

• *THE QUEST FOR A SURROGATE*

Once a couple does decide that they are emotionally ready to use a surrogate, their main problem is how to find one. It is much easier to find someone who is willing to spend a few minutes donating sperm than someone who will make a nine-month loan of her womb. "Realistically, if you wanted to fairly compensate a woman for her time as a surrogate mother, the fee would be phenomenal," declares Katie Brophy, a Louisville attorney who arranges for surrogate parenting on behalf of men whose wives are sterile. "A man who donates sperm anonymously receives twenty five dollars for fifteen minutes of his time, with no risk to himself physically or psychologically. A surrogate is pregnant twenty-four hours a day for nine months."

Because of the difficulty in locating a surrogate, and the potential cost of $5,000 to $25,000 for paying one, some couples turn to women they know to serve as surrogates. One thirty-year-old woman on the East Coast gave birth to a child for her sister.

Family involvement goes even further for a husband and wife who are both infertile. Since they would like to have a child who is genetically related to them, they have recruited his sister and her brother to take part in the process. Her brother will provide the sperm to inseminate his sister, who will bear the child to turn over to the couple.

It is a relief initially to have someone you know and trust serve as surrogate, but it can also be an emotional time bomb. An infertile woman whose sister offers to carry the child should ask herself, How will I feel when the child I am adopting runs into his or her "real" mother at family gatherings? Will I be able to handle my feelings about this special bond my sister and my husband will seem to have (whether they admit any special feeling or not)?

If you ask a friend or relative to bear a child for you, be careful not to pressure her and be sensitive to how such an arrangement would affect her life. In Europe, an infertile woman named Magali begged her twin sister, Christine, for years to bear a child for her. In 1982, Christine was inseminated with the sperm of Magali's husband. Christine's husband left her and their two children, and Christine reports that the arrangement has destroyed her life. She told *Elle* magazine that she carried a child for Magali "to free myself from her."

Deciding to have a woman you know carry the child can work out but it takes some careful emotional discussion and planning before the process begins. Debbie and George's solution of their fertility problem was unique. Since the birth of their child, Sue has lived with them and, a few years ago, bore another child for them.

Debbie, George, and Sue have come through all of this with a very special type of friendship. But there were many issues and hurt feelings between them and negative attitudes from outsiders that had to be worked out along the way. Couples planning to have a surrogate carry a child for them should try to anticipate these potential problems—and talk over their feelings and decide on the best reaction.

If you have no sister or friend who will serve as a surrogate for personal reasons or if you have rejected the offer of a close friend or relative because it could be too emotionally troublesome, you will be faced with the problem of tracking down a surrogate. Oddly enough, you may be able to find one in the classifieds. A Washington surrogate, for example, advertises that she is available to bear a child for an infertile couple for $15,000. You might send out letters to friends, relatives, former classmates, and co-workers asking them to let you know if they learn of anyone willing to be a surrogate. (This sort of letter chain has been useful for couples who wish to find children for private adoption.) You may even advertise yourself in the city newspaper or in a campus publication. Sperm donors are often found via university dailies; at least a few surrogates who have come forward thus far are students wanting money for medical school or law school tuition.

Perhaps there is even someone you know personally who would agree to be a surrogate for a fee. Jane and John asked John's secretary Mary if she would serve as a surrogate for them. Before attempting a pregnancy, though, they approached the Michigan courts to determine whether they can pay Mary $5,000 for her services.

Another way to reach a surrogate is through a doctor or lawyer. Several years ago, a couple with twelve years of infertility problems, who had undergone several operations, approached Dr. William Karow. They asked whether he would consider artificially inseminating a woman with the husband's sperm so that they could adopt the child. "You find the surrogate and then we'll talk about it," he told them.

"But how do we find the surrogate?" they asked.

"I suppose you could advertise in the Los Angeles *Times*," replied Karow. At first, according to Karow, the newspaper refused to take the ad. "Go back and tell the newspaper more about yourself and why you want to do this," suggested Karow. Eventually, the ad was placed, a surrogate located, and Karow performed the insemination.

"Soon I had a pregnant surrogate on my hands and I wasn't quite sure what to do with her," recalls Karow. "I knew this was apt to be of major significance, yet there were no specific laws on it. So I formed a foundation to examine all the issues involved." Karow also joined with two lawyers, William Handel and Bernard Sherwyn, and a psychologist to handle the many practical aspects of surrogate motherhood.

Thus, the request from an infertile couple led Karow to form one of the country's initial surrogate parenting centers, in Los Angeles. Similar visits from a couple in the Midwest prompted Noel Keane to begin a career as a matchmaker between couples and surrogates; and Richard Levin, to form Surrogate Parenting Associates, Inc. in Louisville. Soon after, Philadelphia attorney Burton Satzberg, along with gynecologist Michael Birnbaum and clinical psychologist Howard Adelman, founded Surrogate Mothering, Ltd.

Now the ranks of the surrogate centers are swelling. Katie Brophy, who originally worked with Levin, formed her own service. A number of women who were turned down as surrogates by existing programs opened their own. A social worker in Topeka, Kansas, formed a surrogate program known as the Hagar Institute. Several surrogates who delivered babies as part of existing programs are now planning to open services of their own.

Katie Brophy expresses concern about the rash of surrogate centers opening. "Anyone can set up a surrogate center," she warns. She feels that couples are safer to consult centers run by doctors and lawyers. "There's an added safeguard when professionals are involved since individuals who are not professionals are not bound by the same standards of ethical or professional liability."

Your cost for using a surrogate service will be considerable— generally around $20,000. That covers payment of the surrogate, legal fees, medical fees, and counseling fees. Sometimes part of the cost can be recovered through insurance. The surrogate might have her own insurance to cover her medical costs. You might also ask your employer whether your health insurance covers adoptions. One Chicago woman who adopted a baby privately learned that her company would pay $4,000 of her adoption-related costs.

The surrogate process differs radically from center to center across the country. There are variations in the means of choosing surrogates, the type of contact (if any) the couple and surrogate have, and the safeguards to protect the rights of the couple and the surrogate. You should be well informed about all your options so that you can choose the one with which you will feel most comfortable. Even if you choose a particular program because of its geographic proximity, you should be aware of how the other centers operate so that you can make suggestions about how you would like to proceed at each step.

In choosing a program, great care must be taken so that you work with people you can trust. Some doctors, psychologists, lawyers, and other intermediaries are more concerned with making money through arranging for surrogates than with looking after the best interests of the couple who are their clients. If the center you choose has a team of professionals working on the surrogate arrangements, ask to meet the entire group (for example, the lawyer and the psychologist or other counselor). These people will be choosing the woman who will bear your child. They will be your agents in dealing with the surrogate, so any complaints she has about how they treat her may transfer into hostility toward you. It is critical that you feel comfortable with all the professionals involved. You should also ask how the surrogate will be chosen, what sort of psychological and medical screening will be done, what type of counseling will be available to the surrogate as the pregnancy proceeds, and what legal rights and responsibilities you, your spouse, and the surrogate and her spouse have at each stage of the process.

• *WHO BECOMES A SURROGATE?*

Less than a decade ago, no one had even heard of the term surrogate mother. When the concept was suggested, biologist and ethicist Leon Kass wrote in the *Journal of the American Medical Association* that only prostitutes would serve as surrogates. Attorney Angela Holder suggested in 1977 that perhaps only very poor women would be surrogates. She felt the health of the child would be endangered by a poor surrogate carrier suffering from malnutrition and anemia.

"When we started looking for surrogates, we anticipated that a low class of people would apply, motivated strictly by the economic incentive," says Karow. "Instead we found just the opposite to be true. We found that their reasons for wanting to do this are legitimate, wholesome, and thought through thoroughly. Many have friends or a sister with a long history of infertility or lost children."

What motivates a woman to become a surrogate? Although 80 percent of the surrogates who come forth say they would not proceed without payment, the reasons a woman will choose this unique form of employment are varied and complex. Philip Parker, a practicing psychiatrist and clinical instructor at Wayne State University School of Medicine in Detroit, interviewed over two hundred surrogates. He found that about one third had voluntarily aborted or given up a child in the past. Women who feel guilty about these past experiences, according to Parker, "become surrogates in order to repeat and master that prior experience."

"One surrogate applicant was made to give up a child when she was thirteen," Parker reports. "She wanted to master and do it again and give up the child because she *wanted* to this time. Another felt guilty about 'murdering' a child by having an abortion years earlier, so she wanted to give life to a child."

Other women enter into surrogate arrangements because they enjoy being pregnant. "Many say they would like to be pregnant their whole lives," states Parker. "They just don't want to rear children their whole lives." For example, nineteen-year-old Corinne Appleyard, who served as a surrogate for George and Sheila Syrkowski, claims that she feels more energy when she's pregnant. Surrogate Elizabeth Kane once remarked, "I have babies so easily. They just pop out."

Another strong thread that runs throughout surrogates' motivation is, as Karow pointed out, a close association with an infertile couple. The surrogate may have a close friend or relative who cannot conceive. In fact, she may have been raised by an infertile couple. Nina Kellogg, a California psychologist, found that nearly 20 percent of the surrogates she interviewed were adopted. "They see surrogating as a way of saying thank you to their own parents for their happy homes," remarks Kellogg.

Sometimes the surrogate herself may have had a fertility problem in the past. "Some surrogates adopted their first child and then were able to have a second child naturally," notes Howard Adelman, who points out that such women can understand what the couple is going through. At least two women have become surrogate mothers to avert infertility. "They are doing it because they have endometriosis and their physicians told them they should get pregnant," says Parker.

Whatever compels women to join the surrogate ranks, the demographic profile of the surrogate is as follows. The average age, according to Dr. Parker, is twenty-five. Half the women are married, one-quarter divorced and one-quarter single. Half are Catholic, half Protestant. Over half have high school degrees and about 10 percent have bachelors degrees. Of the first fifty surrogates Parker interviewed, 40 percent were unemployed and the other 60 percent had household incomes of $6,000 to $55,000. As surrogate parenting gets more widespread, though, Parker is finding that more middle class women are applying.

• *CHOOSING A SURROGATE*

When you choose a surrogate, you will be making a monumental decision second only, perhaps, to your choice of a spouse. But unlike the choice of a mate, you won't have months or years to get to know a surrogate mother before you enter this unique relationship. You may have to decide rapidly, on the basis of a two-page written application, sometimes a photo, or perhaps a brief meeting.

Couples who use surrogates apply varied selection criteria. For Dan and Ellen, Karen seemed to be a perfect surrogate because she resembled Ellen. Another couple chose a surrogate because her own children were such darlings. Still other couples have numerous requirements for surrogates, asking them to take IQ tests and aptitude tests before employing them. A single man who wanted a surrogate asked for one who combined the looks of Brigitte Bardot with the brains of Eleanor Roosevelt.

Los Angeles attorney William Handel rejects couples if he thinks they are attempting to create a superchild, because he feels they may not be happy if their child does not turn out exactly as planned. Already, one couple who chose a particular surrogate because of her blonde hair was disappointed when the baby turned out to have brown hair. "I've turned down couples who said, 'We want someone five feet three inches tall with an I.Q. of one hundred and fifty-six,'" reports Handel. "I don't want to be accused of playing eugenics. I explain to couples that we can try for a surrogate who looks reasonably close to you, is emotionally stable and physically healthy. If you want to go beyond that, this is not the office."

• *HOW SURROGATES CHOOSE COUPLES*

When surrogate applicant Karen first met Dan and Ellen in the attorney's office, she recalls, "It was like a mutual employment interview." The screening process goes both ways; the couples are not only scrutinizing but being scrutinized. Many surrogates have their own criteria about what they will—or will not—accept in a couple.

One surrogate searched for a couple who would offer a good Christian home life. According to Parker's study, about one half of the surrogates want assurances that they will be carrying a child for an infertile married woman, not a single man or a woman who is using them for convenience,

In her first surrogate pregnancy, Carol Pavek asked that the husband not be over six feet tall—she did not want a big baby. After that baby was born on February 5, 1981, and successfully adopted by the couple, Pavek was swamped with requests from other couples who wanted her to serve as a surrogate. For various reasons, she has turned down about two hundred couples who have called her.

"I want to feel that I've personally selected a good home for my baby," she says. "I don't want to worry for the next eighteen years whether the couple is financially and emotionally stable."

Carol has refused to serve as a surrogate for a couple who wanted a child just because they needed an heir, and for a couple who she thought would not spend enough recreational time with the child. She has also turned down couples who already have children through adoption or previous marriages.

Her first surrogate experience also gave her ideas about what to request to protect herself and the child in subsequent surrogate pregnancies.

"I certainly want life insurance this time," she remarks, "and I want decision-making power over the baby's medical care for the first twenty-four hours." The latter requirement will ensure that doctors know where to turn in case they need consent for emergency medical services to the child and will allow her to refuse tests on the baby that she, as a midwife, feels are unnecessary.

Some surrogate parenting programs have specific criteria about the type of people they will match with a surrogate. "Basically we're looking for whether the couple has come to terms psychologically with infertility," says Los Angeles psychologist Arlene Westley. "If not, what they need is therapy, not a baby."

A number of programs allow only married couples with infertility problems to use the service. "We turn down everybody but infertile couples," says William Handel. "It's not a moral decision, but a policy decision. Morally I'm in favor of anyone who wants children having them. But we have a responsibility. We have to make surrogate parenting as palatable to the general public as possible. We are trying to get legislation passed."

Noel Keane, in contrast, appears to have no limits on whom he matches with a surrogate. He has been willing to find a surrogate for a single man and even for a single woman, a university professor who did not want a pregnancy to interfere with her chance of getting tenure. In an even more controversial move, Keane has agreed to represent a man who wants a surrogate to use his sperm to conceive a son for him. The man has no interest in rearing the child. Rather, he will establish a $20,000 trust fund for the boy, leave the child in the care of the surrogate and her husband, and seek an unclelike relationship with the child. Many infertile couples who wish to use a surrogate shudder when they hear of such unorthodox parenting arrangements, feeling that they give the whole procedure a bad name.

• *KEEPING YOUR PROMISES*

The most important issue for both sides of any surrogate arrangement is whether each feels the other side will keep its promises. From the couple's point of view, some predictions about the surrogate must be made to try to ensure that the woman will stand by her promise to turn over the child. After years of infertility treatments and maybe even years of trying to find the right surrogate, you would not want to have your hopes dashed nine months later when the surrogate decides to keep the child.

Such was the case of James and Bjorna Noyes of Rochester, New York. Unable to have their own child, they were one of the many couples who asked Noel Keane to find a surrogate for them. Around that same time, Nisa Bhimani, a twenty-nine-year-old Arcadia, California, woman contacted Keane. She had read about him in an article in the *Star,* a tabloid newspaper sold in supermarkets, and was willing to volunteer to be a surrogate for no charge beyond her medical expenses.

Keane and the Noyeses felt they had found the perfect situation.

A simple twelve-line "statement of understanding" was drawn up to outline the arrangement and make clear that "actual and legal custody of the child" would go to the Noyeses. Nisa was inseminated twice with James' sperm (the first one did not "take") and when Nisa announced she was pregnant, the Noyeses were thrilled. The pregnancy progressed beautifully, and the Noyeses readied their life for the arrival of the child.

As the birth approached, Bhimani decided that she wanted to keep the child. James Noyes brought suit to win custody, but California law, which said that a man who donates semen to a woman other than his wife is "not the natural father of the child thereby conceived," presented what appeared to be an insurmountable barrier. Noyes withdrew his custody suit just minutes before it was to be heard and Bhimani got to keep the child.

How can a couple ensure that something like this will not happen to them? In truth, there are no guarantees. Many professionals who work in this area, however, do have rules of thumb about what type of surrogate they think would not be as likely to have second thoughts and want to keep the child.

"For me, it is crucial that the surrogate has already had children of her own," mentions one doctor. "Then she will realize exactly what she is getting into and have a better idea of whether she will be able to go through the pregnancy and then give the child up."

Not all experts follow these guidelines. Noel Keane has asked at least one single, childless surrogate to participate in the program. "She always gets involved in causes," comments her mother.

And, as the Bhimani case demonstrates, previous motherhood is not enough to assure that a surrogate will actually abide by her contract and turn over the child. A Columbus, Ohio, woman had given birth to three beautiful girls of her own before she agreed to be inseminated and serve as a surrogate. But when the baby arrived—a boy—the surrogate decided to keep him to round out her family. She named the child after her husband, even though he had not participated in the boy's conception.

• *WHAT TO LOOK FOR IN A SURROGATE MOTHER*

When trying to find a surrogate who will not disappoint you by trying to keep the child, you should find out what the woman's motives are for becoming a surrogate. A woman who wants to be a surrogate because pregnancy makes her feel special and womanly may decide to keep the child because motherhood does the same thing for her. A woman whose sole motive is "cause" oriented may not have the commitment to continue with the pregnancy and may decide to abort a fetus a few months into the pregnancy, when a new cause catches her fancy.

Let us examine the motives of the surrogates in a few cases where the pregnancy and adoption did go as planned.

Carol Pavek is a midwife in Amarillo, Texas. Because of her commitment to midwifery, Carol and her husband, Rick, decided that she wanted to have her own child at home. Complications arose during labor, however, and, much to Carol's disappointment, she had to give birth at a hospital. Carol wanted to try another home birth but she and Rick did not feel that they could afford another child.

Then Carol saw Keane on a television show and decided that serving as a surrogate would allow her to do something worthwhile for another couple. "When I told my husband I was thinking about becoming a surrogate, he was very encouraging," says Carol. "In fact, he put the paper and pen in my hand to write to Noel Keane."

Elizabeth Kane was responding to a newspaper ad when she called Richard Levin of the Surrogate Parenting Associates to offer her services. She was thirty-seven years old with three children of her own, and had enjoyed her pregnancies. After the births of their children, however, her husband had undergone a vasectomy.

In volunteering to become a surrogate mother, Kane claims to have been motivated by both a desire to be pregnant again and to share her body with the infertile couple. It may be difficult to understand how a surrogate mother would go through the morning sickness of pregnancy, the expansion of her body, the growing bond with the child within her, and the pain of childbirth only to give the child up. But as Parker has pointed out, a number of women find pleasure just in being pregnant. "It gives some women a feeling of power," he explains. "They are creating new life, something no man can do. Pregnancy is the last word in femininity."

Michigan Attorney General Frank Kelley, who objects to surrogate mothering, is suspicious of any woman who gives totally altruistic motives for her desire to become a surrogate mother. Very few women would be willing to do it sheerly for "the joy of making two strangers happy," claims Kelley. That's why a fee is paid— to get the surrogate to "conceive a child she would not normally want to conceive, carry for nine months a child she would not normally want to carry, give birth to a child she would not normally want to give birth to. Then, because of this monetary reward, she relinquishes her parental rights to the child that she bore."

In fact, money and fame may have actually been Kane's real motives for becoming a surrogate. Her fee was reportedly between $5,000 and $10,000 and she seems to revel in the appearances she has made in the mass media. One reason why Kane, like Pavek, was such a good candidate for surrogate parenting, though, was the stability of her home life.

Both Pavek and Kane already had active family lives of their own—with children and husbands they cared very much about. The surrogate parenting decision was a *family* decision for both; their husbands were encouraging about their taking on this new responsibility. In general, Kane and Pavek were happy with their lives and had a stable routine with husband and family to return to once the pregnancy ended and they turned over the baby to the contracting couple.

This has been true in other successful surrogate situations. Madona Patterson's husband, John, pampered her during her surrogate pregnancy, just as he had when she was pregnant with their four children. "He was very caring," reflects Madona, "even driving forty miles in the middle of the night to find kiwis when I had a taste for them."

Contrast that stability and joint decision-making to the home life of Nisa Bhimani, the surrogate who went to court to keep the child. She was alone, raising three children on her own when she decided to become a surrogate. Five years earlier, while she was pregnant with her first child, her husband apparently had killed himself.

While Pavek and Kane did not want to change their lives, but instead saw surrogate parenting as something they could do in addition to their own comforting routines, Bhimani did not have a similar support system. Almost from the beginning, she had doubts. After a first insemination attempt failed, she did not really want to go ahead. When sperm from James Noyes arrived again, air freight, she decided she was obligated to go through with another attempt, all the time subconsciously wishing it wouldn't "take." When she did become pregnant, however, she apparently decided that she could not relinquish the baby and decided to keep the child for herself.

Some potential surrogates try to find comfort and a new life through surrogate parenting. Such motivations can be problematic. When a woman seeks a new life through surrogate mothering, she may not be able to get it from the "surrogate" part because being a surrogate is temporary—a mere nine months. So, instead, she may try to get it from the "mothering" part by keeping the child.

• *WHAT TYPE OF SCREENING SHOULD BE DONE?*

Other than the general observation that a surrogate mother should have a support system to make the process easier, it is hard to tell what makes a good surrogate. When Noel Keane first started matching couples and surrogates, he really had no idea what to look for. Consequently, he committed several egregious errors. Among his first surrogates was an alcoholic woman who threatened midpregnancy to move out of state and keep the child. She tried to extort money from the couple and, because of her drinking problem, the baby was born with fetal alcohol syndrome. To be fair, though, it is not always the surrogate who is the potential troublemaker. One surrogate went to visit the couple who would be using her. The first evening, the wife artificially inseminated her with the husband's sperm. The second day, the wife left for work and the husband asked the surrogate, "Why don't we do it the natural way?" The embarrassed and upset surrogate immediately called a cab for the airport.

As surrogate parenting becomes more widespread, the centers have begun to employ professionals, such as psychiatrists and psychologists, to evaluate surrogates. If you use a center, ask to meet the member of the team who has prime responsibility for screening the surrogate. Make sure that he or she is using reasonable criteria to choose or eliminate surrogates.

Philip Parker, who interviews the women who apply to Noel Keane, feels that so little is known about surrogates that it is impossible for him to eliminate anyone. "I wouldn't know what a good surrogate is," acknowledges Parker. "For all we know, the more disturbed she is the better." Parker feels that his role is not to pick surrogates, but to help them understand themselves and make their own decisions about whether they should participate as a surrogate.

Howard Adelman, who works with the surrogate program in Philadelphia, disagrees with Parker's approach. "I turn surrogates down," maintains Adelman. "I eliminate them if they show depression or anxiety or if they are unreliable. I do a lot of cross-examining of surrogates to be ultra careful."

Adelman worries about letting any surrogate in the program if he has any doubt about her ability to give up the child. In another state, a woman had become a surrogate because she hoped her lover would see how happy she was pregnant and ask her to marry him. "I would have turned that woman down," insists Adelman. "I'd want to know, why is the need there? If she wants to be a surrogate to get somebody, then she might try to use the child to get somebody, too."

Even if you can get over the hurdle of finding a surrogate who agrees to bear and relinquish the child, other screening is necessary before you proceed. The surrogate should undergo medical tests to determine that she is in good health and is likely to bear a healthy child. You may wish to have genetic screening of the surrogate to learn whether she is likely to pass on a serious defect to the child. It is not enough to take the surrogate's word that she is healthy. "The lure of $10,000 might get the surrogate to conceal a genetic defect," law professor Frederica Lombard of Wayne State University told the audience of a surrogate mother conference.

Medical testing of the surrogate is particularly important for couples in which the husband is the carrier of a recessive defect. Such screening can avert the tragedy that has occasionally occurred with artificial insemination, where donors unwittingly (or even perhaps knowingly) have sold semen that carries a genetic defect, such as Tay-Sachs trait. In such cases, the couple have found that the child for whom they longed for so many years will die before he or she even reaches school age.

In addition to the medical testing, an assessment must be made of the surrogate's lifestyle to see whether any stresses she is under or habits she has could adversely affect the child who is growing in her womb. A woman who drinks or smokes excessively, although willing to be a surrogate, would not prove to be the best incubator for a child.

• HOW MUCH CONTACT SHOULD YOU HAVE WITH THE SURROGATE?

Even if you have used a surrogate center to evaluate women for you, the doctor, lawyer, or psychologist involved will probably ask you to make the final choice. The process of choice can differ radically from that of artificial insemination. When it is the man who is infertile and artificial insemination is being used on his wife, the couple tell their doctor what sort of traits they would like the donor to have. Most often, they want a donor who looks like the husband, but other traits of the donor—intelligence, athletic skills, religion—might also be important. The doctor generally calls upon a donor who has those traits. Throughout the process, the donor remains anonymous. The couple never see him, talk to him, or learn his identity.

Contrast this with the surrogate mother situation, where there is often contact between the couple and the woman who will carry their child. At Levin's program, the couple can look at pictures of potential surrogates in order to choose one. This direct approach has potential pitfalls: it may put too much emphasis on the surrogate's appearance, rather than her medical and psychological suitability, and it may cause the husband to start fantasizing about the woman who will bear his child.

For some couples, the contact with the surrogate is even more intimate than viewing her picture. Less than a week after midwife Carol Pavek wrote to Noel Keane, she received a phone call from two of his clients, a California couple who were searching for a surrogate. A week later, the couple flew to Texas to meet her. The artificial insemination took place in Pavek's home during that visit. The couple went into one bedroom of the Pavek home with a paper cup and the wife came out with a sample of her husband's semen in the cup. Because of Pavek's midwife training, she felt capable of inseminating herself (rather than calling in a doctor). She did so using a drugstore syringe.

Before rushing in to meet the woman who will carry your child, think carefully about whether it is really necessary. Surrogate Mothering, Ltd. in Philadelphia, operates successfully without any contact between couples and surrogates. The founders of that program feel it causes less emotional stress for all involved to remain anonymous. ("Besides," jokes Burton Satzberg, "then the surrogate can think she is carrying Robert Redford's child instead of the child of a little bald man with a mustache.") The Philadelphia program gives each couple the profiles of three different surrogates to choose from. If the surrogate they pick miscarries, the couple can select from a group of three more.

In the Los Angeles program run by William Handel, Bernard Sherwyn, and William Karow, the surrogate and couple meet only once, on a first-name basis. "These sessions in which the couple and surrogate meet are crucial to what I call the 'bonding process,'" notes Nina Kellogg. "During this time the surrogate usually 'bonds' with the couple, particularly to the woman she is bearing the child for. After the initial uneasiness is over, everyone starts seeking out similarities in each other and the couple often shares with the surrogate what they have gone through with their infertility problem. Through this meeting, the surrogate achieves the full realization that the child she will carry is not hers but the couple's. She realizes her specialness and that she controls their potential destiny as a family."

Apparently this bonding worked in the case of Karen, who became pregnant as a surrogate for Dan and Ellen. When, a few months into the pregnancy, Karen suffered a miscarriage, she was more concerned about Dan and Ellen than herself. "I felt terrible for them, as if I got their hopes up and dashed them," says Karen. Her first words after the miscarriage were, "Will Dan and Ellen be all right?"

Beyond deciding whether you want to have an initial first-name meeting with the surrogate, you may face the question of whether to let yourself be identified fully to the surrogate or even visit or call each other occasionally during the pregnancy. Personal contact with the surrogate during the pregnancy can be exciting. When the surrogate feels the baby's first kick, the couple can immediately share it. But the pleasure that the personal contact brings in those nine months may be a high price to pay for the problems it could cause in the long run. The value of anonymous surrogate mothering, like anonymous artificial insemination, comes later. When anonymity is retained, the couple have a better chance of developing their own strong relationship with the child.

Although there may be a great temptation to get close to the surrogate, think carefully about whether that will really be best for you. If you do not get involved, the surrogate will not become a part of the "family." She can then be thought of—as Elizabeth Kane tried to think of herself—as a "human incubator." It may seem a bit cruel to refer to another human being like that, particularly one who is sharing her body with a couple (whether for a fee or not) to ensure that they have a child. But unless the surrogate is chosen particularly because of her relationship with the couple (relative, friend), it may be in the best interests of the couple to avoid contact with the surrogate. In this way, they will not feel obligated to "share" the child with her in any way and the child will have a chance to grow up in as normal a family as possible, with the chance of having a strong sense that the couple are his or her parents.

As a middle ground between total lack of contact and an attempt to develop a friendship, you could communicate with the surrogate through the attorney, doctor, or other intermediary (for example, through letters that do not reveal your full name or other identifying information). This may help the peace of mind of both you and the surrogate—so neither party feels the other will renege.

"In our program, the couple and surrogate send each other letters," observes Beth Bridgman of the Hagar Institute. "They address each other as 'Dear Friend' or with nicknames they've created. The letters help the couple and surrogate to bond to each other."

In addition to deciding whether you want to meet the surrogate at the interview stage or during the pregnancy, you will have to ask yourselves whether you want to be present at the birth.

When surrogate Elizabeth Kane gave birth, the couple was in the delivery room with her. The baby was given right to the adoptive mother instead of to Elizabeth.

At first she held him gingerly.

"Does he feel like your son?" Elizabeth asked.

"No," she replied.

"But," Elizabeth recounted later, "an hour later she was holding and kissing him all over and if anyone had come in the room they'd have no doubt about the fact that these two belonged together."

Couples vary in the arrangements they make with the surrogate as to whether she can visit, touch, or feed the baby in the hospital. One couple let the surrogate keep the baby for a week to breast-feed since they felt it would be best for the health of the child.

"Inviting the adopting mother to the delivery room is sometimes done today even in some traditional private adoptions," reports Carol Pavek. "Seconds after birth the pink squealy baby is put directly on the adoptive mother's belly so that they may bond."

Being in the delivery room can allow the couple to share the joy of their child's birth, yet anonymity can be maintained. The surgical masks, caps, and scrubsuits the couple wear conceal their identity.

One infertile couple plans a unique approach to the birth of their child. At the surrogate's request, the husband, an obstetrician, and his infertile wife will preside over the child's home birth.

• *THE EMOTIONAL ASPECTS OF THE SURROGATE PROCESS*

The joy of creating a child through surrogate motherhood is incredible. One six-foot-tall husband burst into tears when his child entered the world through the womb of a surrogate. After nineteen years of infertility, he and his wife had finally found the child they longed for.

Before couples reach the exhilarating point of holding their own child in their arms, however, they go through an emotional barrage. Early in the procedure, the wife may feel awkward and left out. "There need to be tactics to make the adoptive mother more involved," Detroit psychiatrist Lawrence Tourkow told the audience at a surrogate mother conference. "She seems to be the alien who has to look for a place to register."

Throughout the surrogate pregnancy, both the husband and his infertile wife may have fears about losing the child, wondering if the surrogate will keep him or her. Thus the couple may be concerned about not only their own feelings but also the emotions that the surrogate is experiencing and how they will affect her relationship with the child. The surrogate, like the couple, goes through a range of emotions during the pregnancy.

When the baby first begins to move inside the surrogate, comments Philip Parker, "she experiences the pregnancy in a more striking manner. The surrogate has feelings at that time of anticipated sadness." The surrogate must begin to erect an emotional barrier at that time so that she experiences the child not as hers but as the child of the couple.

Because surrogate motherhood is launching women into unchartered emotional territory, it is important to learn whether the woman who will carry your child can cope with the changing emotions. Find out whether the woman has a husband, lover, or another person in her life who is supportive of her decision and will help her through the process. If you are working through a surrogate program, ask whether they provide counseling services for the surrogate during and after the pregnancy. Women recruited by Surrogate Mothering, Ltd., in Philadelphia, go through monthly individualized counseling. Parker runs group counseling sessions for surrogates in Michigan, as does the Columbus, Ohio, program and the Los Angeles program.

The most emotionally volatile time for the surrogate—right after the birth—is the period during which she gets the least help. All attention centers on the couple.

Even the hospital staff can be insensitive to the surrogate's feelings. When she was being wheeled back to her room after an exhausting labor and birth, surrogate Julie Gallimore was asked by a nurse, "I know this is a bad time to ask, but why did you decide to give up your baby for money?"

"Don't put us back on the shelf after the birth," Elizabeth Kane told a group of infertile couples in the process of considering or using surrogates. "We're not disposable wombs. Whether a surrogate or the mother of a stillborn, there's still a need to say good-bye."

"The books and movies about surrogate mothering all end with the delivery," charges Julie Gallimore, "but we need emotional support even after the birth. I was sailing through pregnancy and was unprepared for the feeling I had after I came home from the hospital."

Because of the uncertain legal status of surrogate motherhood, some lawyers tell the surrogate she must take the baby home from the hospital and then turn it over to the couple later. This can be emotionally traumatic for the surrogate. "An exchange in a parking lot or an attorney's office is not adequate to erase the memory of leaving the hospital with the baby," cautions Gallimore.

Another surrogate feels emotionally brutalized by the way her exchange was handled. As a surrogate for a single man, she has the nagging feeling that she is still the mother. She had to stay in the hospital an extra day solely because the father had to give a speech and could not pick up the baby.

"This is something I'll have to handle for the rest of my life," says Gallimore about her surrogate pregnancy. "I only ask that they take care of me for the couple months after the delivery."

Such caretaking could take the form of having counseling available for the surrogate in the weeks or months after the baby is born. "There are striking psychological consequences to surrogate motherhood," observes Parker, "After the surrogate gives birth, there is generally a period of grief and mourning that lasts from four to six weeks. At that time the surrogate may experience crying and difficulty sleeping, at least in the short run. This needs to be followed up further, particularly on the birth date of the child."

• *THE SOCIAL ASPECTS OF THE SURROGATE PROCESS*

When Elizabeth Kane was resting on the examination table after her insemination took place, her mind bubbled with thoughts. She thought about how she was creating what she called a "gift of love" for the infertile couple. She thought about how good it was that her husband, initially skeptical about the idea, had come around. Now he had promised to help her through childbirth, doing Lamaze coaching. She felt so happy about what she was doing that it never dawned on her that other people might not also view favorably her acting as a surrogate. During her ten minutes of quiet contemplation on the examining table, she hardly imagined the harassment and bitterness she would encounter from family, neighbors, and friends.

For some reason, when an infertile couple uses a surrogate, it seems as if everyone in the world feels they have a right to comment on it. This is also a difference between surrogate parenting and artificial insemination. When the husband is infertile and his wife undergoes artificial insemination, her pregnancy is viewed as natural by neighbors and family members who may not even know of the husband's infertility.

When the wife is sterile and the couple uses a surrogate, however, observers will easily know something is unusual. The wife will not be visibly pregnant before the arrival of the couple's child.

Meanwhile, the waistline will be expanding on the surrogate—who may be unmarried or, like Elizabeth Kane, married to a man who friends and relatives know has undergone a vasectomy.

Every participant in the surrogate triangle must make a decision about what and how much he or she will tell observers. One couple has decorated a nursery while they wait for a successful insemination of the woman who has agreed to be their surrogate. When they learn that the surrogate is pregnant, they plan to open a bottle of champagne and to call friends and relatives to announce they are pregnant.

In many instances, however, when the couple and surrogate have told people about their joint pregnancy, their excitement and joy have not been shared.

Debbie's in-laws have snubbed her and her husband since the couple had their friend Sue give birth to two children for them. They sought religious support, but a priest told them, "There's no sin on your children, but the sin is on you. You've used sperm in another woman's body."

The surrogate, too, may encounter disdain. Elizabeth Kane's parents accused her of giving away their grandchild. Schoolmates taunted Kane's children, calling Kane a baby-seller, and a friend branded her as an adulteress. One twenty-year-old has even more problems. Since she is single, her decision raised eyebrows in her home community in suburban Maryland. She was forced to move out of her parents' home and into an apartment elsewhere.

The opposition to surrogate motherhood concentrates partially on its effect on the surrogate, but more frequently on its effect on the child. Washington, D.C., psychiatrist E. James Lieberman opposes the procedure because he does not think a surrogate can predict how she will feel after she gives up the child. Canadian psychiatrist Thomas Verny opposes surrogate motherhood for another reason. He believes that a fetus within a woman's body is sensitive to the emotions of its mother. If the surrogate distances herself from the child within her, that child may develop psychological problems. Others point out that the child may be harmed since the couple who can afford the expensive surrogate procedure are not necessarily a couple who would make good parents.

The payment aspect of surrogating is particularly troublesome. Vaughn Adams, an assistant professor of philosophy at the University of Detroit, describing the Roman Catholic viewpoint on surrogate motherhood, told the audience of a surrogate conference at Wayne State University, "The fact that there's $10,000 or $20,000 or $5,000 involved is so heinous that I don't want to talk about it."

A Michigan woman who testified at legislative hearings on surrogate parenting, pointed out that "the idea of an exchange of money in connection with surrogate parenting would seem to create an uncomfortable position for the adopted person. I do not believe, for any reason, one can put a price on a human life. As an adoptee, I would find it appalling and insulting to think that my parents had 'bought' me and that my birth mother had accepted money for my life. I would find it uncomfortable to think that a price such as $10,000 was the extent of my worth, and, on the other hand, I would also be concerned with the expectations of me which accompanied the payment of a sum of money."

The distaste people feel about surrogate parenting is sometimes aggravated by the lawyers and doctors involved. One attorney made the process seem like selling puppies. He suggested that if the surrogate had triplets, the couple might agree to let her keep one.

Because of the sentiment against surrogate motherhood, a surrogate might be pressured by family and friends to keep the child. This is another reason why the process of choosing the surrogate is important. She must be able to withstand these pressures.

"If I were donating a kidney no one would be appalled," protested Kane during her surrogate pregnancy, "but because I'm lending one of my ovaries, loaning out my womb to someone, people look at me like I'm a freak. They stop me in the street and say 'How can you give your baby away?' But what they can't realize is that I'm not giving it away, I'm returning the child inside me to its father."

· *SURROGATE MOTHERING AND THE LAW*

Unfortunately, the law is generally no more sympathetic to surrogate mothers than are their neighbors. The law views the woman who bears a child as its natural mother. That is why the baby must be adopted by the couple (or at least the wife of the man) who contracted for it. Yet many states have statutes requiring that all adoptions go through a public agency and prohibiting a mother from accepting money for turning over her child.

When these laws were initially passed, the possibility of surrogate motherhood by artificial insemination was not even considered. They were developed to prevent an already pregnant woman from being talked out of her baby by someone offering to pay her medical expenses and perhaps some additional sum. The lawmakers felt that mere willingness to pay does not guarantee that the new parents would be fit. So these laws were enacted to ensure that more traditional adoption procedures would be followed.

The use of a surrogate mother differs in some important ways from paying a pregnant woman for her child. First, the contract is made before the woman is pregnant, and thus it is less likely that she will be taken advantage of. Moreover, since the adopting father is the natural father, the child is more likely to be given a good home.

In some states the man who provides the sperm may have a difficult time establishing that he is the legal father of the child. When artificial insemination was first being used in the United States, there was a fear that the donor of the semen would be held liable for the costs of raising the child. So some states (California, Colorado, Connecticut, Montana, Nevada, Minnesota, Oregon, Texas, Wisconsin, and Wyoming) passed laws saying that when a man donates sperm for artificial insemination of a woman who is *not* his wife, that donor is *not* the father of the child. Obviously, these laws impede the surrogate mother arrangement, in which the donor of the semen *does* in fact want to be considered the father. Equally troublesome are laws in twenty-two states that make an inseminated woman's husband the legal father if he has consented to the insemination.

A couple considering using a surrogate thus must think of the legal ramifications. Because the acknowledged use of surrogates began only recently and the first court case involving a surrogate mother did not take place until 1980, there are only a handful of lawyers in the country who are well versed in this area.

If you consult your family lawyer, he or she might tell you, "There are no laws on surrogate mothering in this state." That is true since, so far, no state has a law specifically governing the process and only a few states appear to be considering such laws. However, there are a number of other laws that affect the legality of various aspects of the process. For example, the artificial insemination laws (discussed in detail in Chapter Seven) govern the insemination of the surrogate and the adoption laws cover her giving up the child.

If you want a legal opinion about surrogate parenting in your state, it might help to point your lawyer in the right direction by asking about various applicable laws. The lawyer should check to see whether there is a law governing artificial insemination in the state where that process will take place and, if there is, whether that law creates a presumption that the donor is not the legal father.

The lawyer should also check the adoption laws. First, he or she should check to see whether "private" adoption is allowed. If it is not allowed, this could cause problems no matter whether the surrogate is to be paid or not. Second, he or she should check to see whether payment in connection with an adoption is forbidden. For example, in Florida, no payment may be made in connection with an adoption except the medical and living expenses of the mother through pregnancy and thirty days after the birth. Third, he or she should see whether the law provides any sort of waiting period. In Kentucky, where Levin's program is located, for example, the law provides that a woman may not consent to terminate her parental rights or give her child up for adoption until five days after the baby's birth. This gives the mother a cooling-off period to make

228 · NEW CONCEPTIONS

sure her decision is a well-considered one. But it also means that any contract the woman makes before her pregnancy is illegal (since it was made before the waiting period ended). Yet contracts made after the waiting period would also be void since the child already has been born and thus it would be considered to be "child selling."

In addition, the lawyer should look into the family law of the state in which the surrogate lives. In at least twenty-eight states, the husband of any woman who gets pregnant during the marriage is presumed to be the father of the child, and the courts often will not even admit blood tests or other evidence to show that he could not actually have fathered the child. This means that in such states, the surrogate's husband would have rights to the child. The surrogate's husband would be presumed by the law to be the father even if, as in the case of Elizabeth Kane's husband, he had undergone a vasectomy and clearly could not have produced a child. Some attorneys try to avoid this presumption of paternity by using divorced or single women as surrogates.

In addition to these laws covering artificial insemination, adoption, and the rights of the surrogate's husband, other obscure laws might be in effect in your state that could possibly affect a surrogate's contract. For example, some states have antislavery laws that prohibit selling "people." These could be used to prevent a surrogate from accepting a fee to bear a child and turn him or her over to you.

Your chances of legally obtaining a child through surrogate mothering are eased considerably in states that have special stepparent adoption laws. These laws create a streamlined adoption procedure when the biological parents' spouse (i.e., the stepparent) wishes to adopt the child. In the surrogate situation, the biological parent is the man whose sperm is used and the stepparent is his infertile wife.

In states where it is available, the stepparent adoption procedure does away with one or more of the following requirements for adoption—the waiting period, suitability investigation, and the prohibition of payment to the biological mother—in situations where the biological father's wife wishes to adopt the child.

To take advantage of this streamlined approach, the husband who has provided the sperm is often advised to have his name put on the birth certificate as the father (even though the surrogate might actually have a husband of her own). After the child's birth, the surrogate (the child's natural mother) agrees to the adoption of the child by the wife. The wife files for the simple stepparent adoption since she is married to the man listed as the father on the birth certificate.

The complexities of the laws that impinge on surrogate motherhood are illustrated by the court cases in which such arrangements have been under fire. Many couples who have entered into a contract with a surrogate mother or are considering solving their infertility problem in this manner were distressed after learning of the Nisa Bhimani case, in which the surrogate decided to keep her child. The case itself provided no legal precedent, however, since it never got to trial. Instead, the couple who had wanted the child, James and Bjorna Noyes, dropped the suit a few minutes before the trial was scheduled to begin.

Before it was dropped, the case proceeded as follows. Bhimani wrote to the Noyes' lawyer during the pregnancy, saying she had decided to keep the child. James Noyes filed suit seeking custody of the then-unborn child. The judge ordered that blood tests be performed on the baby after its birth and on Noyes to determine whether he was really the father.

Before trial, Bhimani's lawyer had the right to question the Noyes couple. He asked Bjorna why she had been unable to have a child and whether she had been known by any other name. Her answers revealed that Bjorna had lived her youth as a male until, after an operation, she began to live as a female.

The Noyes' attorney said that James had decided not to pursue the lawsuit "because the extraordinary publicity would not allow his child to live a normal life. He feels it is in the best interest of the child."

Actually, the Noyeses and their attorney might have felt that the couple could not have won their case once the fact of Bjorna's sex operation came out, since Bjorna's fitness as a parent would have become an issue if the case had proceeded further.

Another case, this one in Michigan, does not pit the surrogate against the couple, but pits all three against the adoption system. This is the case, mentioned earlier, of the couple who wanted to pay the husband's secretary to be inseminated with the husband's sperm and bear a child for them. Since the Michigan law prohibits payment of money in connection with an adoption, such an arrangement would be illegal in that state.

Not wanting to do something illegal, the couple asked their attorney, Noel Keane, to go into court to challenge the law. In May 1978, Keane filed the case, arguing that the statute was an unconstitutional infringement on the right of privacy of the participants.

In January 1980, the judge rejected Keane's argument, insisting that "the State's interest, expressed in the statute . . . is to prevent commercialism from affecting a mother's decision to execute a consent to the adoption of her child. 'Baby-bartering' is against the public policy of this State."

Keane filed an appeal, charging that "a surrogate mother exercises her choice to become a surrogate, prior to conception, and is, therefore, not subject to the duress and anxiety which commonly attaches to an unexpected or unwanted pregnancy."

Attorneys for the state countered Keane's arguments by claiming that allowing women to be paid to act as surrogates would thrust the court into the role of setting prices for children, perhaps allowing higher compensation for a bright, beautiful surrogate as opposed to a less attractive, less intelligent one.

"The integrity of the court system and the statutory adoption process demands that the court be absolutely prohibited from deciding which individual has a Saks Fifth Avenue price tag and which individual has a K-Mart price tag," argued the attorneys for the state.

The Attorney General of Michigan, Frank J. Kelley, also described to the court the dangers that he thought surrogate motherhood wrought. He argued that without specific legislation in Michigan spelling out the rights and responsibilities of the parties involved in a surrogate motherhood contract, too many things could go wrong. Women might be coerced into serving as surrogates, particularly women like Mary Roe, who was being asked to be a surrogate for her boss. The arrangement might be detrimental to the children when they learned that their natural mother gave them up for money. The lack of a law spelling out how a surrogate arrangement should proceed could lead to conflicting claims by the parties. For example, explained Kelley, the "natural mother might renegotiate the fee by withholding consent to adoption or resist if the probate court reduces the fees to be paid to her [or] . . . resist adoption either before or after it is ordered out of guilt or out of the strong bond which quickly develops between parent and infant." Kelley also criticized the surrogate arrangement since it "would permit John Doe to go outside of matrimony to conceive a child." Kelley further challenged Keane's reference to Mary Roe's role as that of surrogate mother. "This jargon serves to gloss over the fact that Mary Roe is the real mother, and Jane Doe would be a substitute (or surrogate) mother if she were permitted to adopt the child," protested Kelley.

The appeals court in the case ruled that although a couple has a right to use a surrogate, they do not have the right to pay money to the surrogate in exchange for adoption and they cannot expect the court to make the child legally theirs. The Michigan Supreme Court was equally unsympathetic to the Doe's request. As a last resort, Keane attempted to plead the case to the U.S. Supreme Court, but the Supreme Court Justices voted eight to one not to consider the case.

Another case involving surrogate parenting is currently taking place in Kentucky. In Kentucky, as in Michigan, the law forbids accepting money in connection with putting a child up for adoption. To steer clear of that law, Surrogate Parenting Associates worded their contracts so that the mother was paid not to put the child up for adoption but to relinquish her parental rights. The exact wording of the Kentucky law apparently does not address such an arrangement. Once the surrogate has terminated her rights to the child, custody would go to the child's *other* biological parent (the man who wants the child and whose semen was used to inseminate the surrogate). When the natural father gets custody, it would be relatively simple for his wife to file for adoption and become a legal parent of the child as well.

This type of arrangement seemed to be working without a hitch for nearly a year in Kentucky. Then, on January 26, 1981, the Kentucky Attorney General, Steven Beshear, issued an opinion stating that it was the policy of the state to forbid "baby buying." He also said that payment for termination of parental rights, although not addressed specifically in the statute, was not permissible since it was being done with the obvious intent to circumvent the adoption statutes. In any event, he felt a surrogate arrangement made before conception was illegal since a mother cannot legally agree to terminate her parental rights in Kentucky until five days after the baby is born.

Acting upon this opinion, Beshear filed suit to try to close down the Surrogate Parenting Associates altogether. That case is still pending.

In Michigan and Kentucky, in two other cases, the arrangements between two particular couples and their surrogates proceeded without a hitch—the babies are now in physical custody of the couples with the surrogate's blessings. But the couples have not managed to obtain legal custody. Even though all the parties have agreed to the arrangements, the courts view them suspiciously and, in both cases, refused to authorize the adoptions. The laws are just not set up for the surrogate arrangement, said the Kentucky judge; "it is much like trying to fit a square peg in a round hole." The Michigan adoption judge had similar qualms. The babies are thus in legal limbo and the couples are left with the fear that the surrogates might excerise a right to custody in the future.

A surrogate case has also taken place across the ocean. In England, a couple engaged a prostitute to be a surrogate mother. The surrogate was inseminated and gave birth to a child but then refused to relinquish the baby. The disappointed couple tried to induce the surrogate by offering money and a secondhand car. Finally, they offered to give her their house. She still wanted to keep the child. The couple sued and when the matter went to court, the judge granted the prostitute custody. The judge refused to enforce what he felt was a pernicious agreement for the sale of a child.

Surrogate mothering is a legally risky procedure. Attorneys

Handel and Sherwyn bluntly inform clients of the pitfalls, explaining that the procedure may violate the criminal laws with respect to slavery, paying money in connection with an adoption, advertising for adoption, or even conspiracy. They also point out numerous other legal liabilities that might exist. The couple might have to share the child in joint custody with the surrogate. Or the couple might not get custody of the child, yet the husband might still have to pay child support to the surrogate.

"Everyone who enters into this needs to do so with caution," says Wyckoff. When she founded the Association for Surrogate Parenting, Inc., Ohio prosecutors informed her that the process was illegal and she could end up in jail. "The threat is still hanging over me," says Wyckoff. "I never know when they'll come to arrest me. My greatest fear is that my children will be home. I don't want them to see the police take me to jail."

• *PUTTING IT IN WRITING*

You may be wondering how any surrogate arrangements take place with this incredible assortment of laws potentially prohibiting or restricting it. As long as your lawyer is aware of the thicket of legal regulations, he or she can plan the best legal procedure for you to become parents, much as your doctor plans the best medical procedure. Thanks to the possibility of freezing sperm and sending it by airplane for use in an insemination in another state, you can choose a surrogate mother in a state whose laws are more favorable to such an arrangement than are your own.

Despite legal risks, many couples want to use a surrogate. They feel that even if the surrogate arrangement takes place in a state where the laws try to deter it, the law will rarely get involved unless (as in the case of Nisa Bhimani) one of the parties wants to renege on the agreement.

That is why it is important to choose the surrogate carefully, as described earlier. It is also advisable to enter into a detailed contract with the surrogate. In that way, all people involved will know exactly what the surrogate situation entails. Any confusion about what a certain party's rights are, or any doubts about whether the arrangement should be undertaken, can thus be cleared up *before* the pregnancy begins.

Drafting a surrogate contract is extremely complex. "Every time you think you've covered every situation, something else comes up," warns Burton Satzburg. In working with your lawyer to put together a contract, keep in mind that the document should spell out the rights and responsibilities of each party—the husband who will be the natural father, the infertile wife, the surrogate, and the surrogate's husband—at each stage of the process.

For example, such a contract should include the basic agreement that the surrogate agrees to be inseminated with a particular man's sperm, carry the baby, and turn it over after its birth to the man and his wife. If the surrogate is to be paid, the contract should also spell out when she will receive the payments, for example, $1,000 when the pregnancy is confirmed, $1,000 midway through the pregnancy, and $8,000 after the baby has been born. The contract might also provide that the surrogate's husband agrees not to claim that he is the legal father of the child.

The contract could also contain specific provisions to help ensure that the baby is healthy. It could stipulate that the surrogate mother should not smoke, drink, or take drugs (other than on a doctor's recommendation) during the pregnancy. The contracts used by the Los Angeles and Philadelphia programs also require that the surrogate avoid exposure to radiation, toxic chemicals, or communicable illness.

The agreement might also provide that the surrogate must undergo amniocentesis at an appropriate point in the pregnancy. For example, since Elizabeth Kane was an older mother (age thirty-eight), and the chances of giving birth to a Down's syndrome child increase as the mother's age increases, Kane was asked to undergo amniocentesis.

The results in Kane's case showed she was carrying a normal fetus. But what if they had not? That is why a contract should describe the rights of the various parties if the fetus is found to have a genetic defect. It should answer the questions: Must the surrogate abort the child on the couple's request? Must she continue to carry it if the couple decides they want it despite the defect? If she decides to have the genetically defective child, despite the couple's wish that she abort, can she then keep the child herself?

Another variation on the situation might occur if the natural father died before the child was born. The contract should cover whether the surrogate mother would then keep the child, whether the natural father's wife (who would not be genetically related to the child) would be given custody of the child, or whether an altogether different arrangement would ensue. At Surrogate Parenting Associates, for example, if the natural father dies, Levin is given custody of the child until he or she is placed for adoption.

The contract might also make other provisions for the welfare of the surrogate and child. The Surrogate Parenting Associates' contract provides that the natural father must pay for an insurance policy on the life of the surrogate, to remain in effect until six months after the baby's birth. The SPA contract also requires that the natural father take out a policy on his own life, payable in trust to the unborn child.

The contract should also provide for some sort of testing to ensure that the child was actually fathered by the man who contracted for it (the husband of a sterile woman) rather than another man with whom the surrogate made love. For example, the contract could provide that the child must undergo certain blood tests. The contract could also provide that if these tests reveal that the husband of the sterile woman was *not* the father, the surrogate would be required to pay back the money she was given and the couple could choose not to accept the child.

A contract might also provide for anonymity for the various parties. They need not sign the same copies of the contract, so there is no reason that they would have to know each other's names. Beyond that, the contract could provide that the natural father and his wife not try to find out the identity and whereabouts of the surrogate (and vice versa) and that the couple not inform the child of the identity of the surrogate.

In addition, many contracts make an attempt to make sure the process goes smoothly psychologically. They require that the surrogate agree that she "will not form a parent-child relationship" with the child she conceived.

The contract designed by Handel and Sherwyn tries to ensure the child's well-being in the future. It provides that the surrogate must furnish them with any changes of address she makes for eighteen years after the child's birth and must provide medical information. The contract also tries to protect both sides and the child from disturbing publicity by requiring that if a dispute arises and the matter goes to court the parties and attorneys agree to keep it confidential.

A surrogate contract provides valuable guidelines for the conduct of the couple and surrogate. But if a surrogate decides to breach the contract and keep the child, it is highly improbable that a court would enforce the contract. Philadelphia lawyer Burton Satzberg explains to prospective parents that if the surrogate changes her mind, she cannot legally be required to terminate her parental rights. Satzberg believes, however, that a court might be willing to accept the contract as proof of paternity, which would allow the genetic father to bring a custody suit. The issue would then become whether the environment the natural father and his wife could provide would be more in the child's best interest than that which the surrogate could offer. The court would carefully judge the facts of the situation and, as it would in any custody dispute, determine if the child could be better cared for by the father (the man who provided the sperm) or the mother (the surrogate).

William Handel tells each surrogate, "I don't know if we're going to be able to enforce the contract if you decide to keep the child. But the couple has already gone through an enormous amount of grief with their infertility and their surgeries. They've used up their money to pay you. If you decide to keep the child, we'll sue you for intentional infliction of emotional distress. You'll have ruined this couple's life. And we'll make it awfully expensive for you to hold on to the child."

• *SURROGATE MOTHER LEGISLATION*

Contracts provide only a partial solution to the legal dilemmas raised by surrogate motherhood. For couples and surrogates to have the peace of mind they deserve when entering into such an intimate, complex relationship, they need to be protected by new state laws. As of this writing, no state had adopted such a law, but the legislatures in Alabama, Alaska, California, Connecticut, Hawaii, Kansas, Michigan, South Carolina, and Tennessee were preparing to vote on surrogate legislation.

By the time this book is published, such a law may actually have been enacted, perhaps even in your home state. If a state law does exist, try to get a copy from your state legislator or a law library so that you can learn your legal rights and responsibilities.

The laws that have been proposed range from bills completely banning the procedure to those allowing it with no limitation on who uses it or what price is paid to the surrogate. All have a history of controversy.

Michigan legislator Richard Fitzpatrick introduced the first surrogate mother bill in the country in October 1981. He admits that his willingness to propose a law legalizing surrogate motherhood was viewed as strange by his lawmaker colleagues. "It deals with emotional issues, it's related to sex and it's a type of a law that no legislature had previously adopted," acknowledges Fitzpatrick, and thus it was the sort of volatile legislation that most legislators avoid. But Fitzpatrick realized that "surrogates were a fact of life in Michigan" and he was concerned about the lack of protection for the parties involved.

The law he developed spelled out in incredible detail the various parties' rights and responsibilities. "This first bill was very complicated," notes Fitzpatrick. "It paralleled as closely as possible the adoption laws."

Under that proposed law, the couple would file a petition with the court asking for permission to enter into a surrogate arrangement. The court would then order a full investigation of the couple, similar to the home study made in the course of a regular adoption. If the couple passed inspection, the artificial insemination could take place. Six months into the pregnancy, the court would enter an order granting custody to the couple after the child's birth. Fourteen days after the child was born, the child would legally be adopted by the couple.

Under the proposed legislation, the responsibilities of all parties would have to be clearly spelled out in contracts. The bill detailed nineteen provisions a surrogate agreement would have to contain, most of which were already in use in the private surrogate contracts. They included numerous requirements for the surrogate: that she undergo psychiatric, medical, and genetic evaluation; that she follow medical instructions and agree not to smoke cigarettes, drink alcohol, or use illegal or nonprescription drugs; that she not abort unless it is necessary for her health or the child is abnormal. The natural father would be required to undergo genetic and medical evaluations, which would include venereal disease testing before each insemination. He and his wife could terminate the contract if the surrogate did not become pregnant within a reasonable time. The legislation provided for several rare but important occurrences. The couple would be responsible for any child born with a congenital abnormality. If either spouse died before the child's birth, the other could still get custody of the child. If both died, the surrogate would still be paid and she would have the choice of keeping the child or putting him or her up for adoption. The maximum fee allowable for a surrogate under the law would be $10,000.

Although Fitzpatrick's proposed law covered virtually all aspects of the surrogate arrangement, it engendered lots of criticism. "When we had hearings on it," says Fitzpatrick, "people began to get hung up on the details. One of the big battles was over the $10,000 limit. In the movie *Paternity*, Burt Reynolds paid $40,000 to the surrogate. For many infertile couples, they'd pay well over $10,000."

Surrogate Carol Pavek was furious about the $10,000 limit. Although she herself had charged no fee the first time she was a surrogate, she argued that the legislature should not limit the compensation. "Why should they set a financial limit? Either payment is legal or it's not," Pavek maintains.

"Instead of setting limits on what a surrogate can get paid, they should set a limit for what psychiatrists, attorneys, and medical doctors can get," she continues. "After all, there is a ceiling on attorneys' fees for adoption. And once you get a precedent set, it shouldn't be that tough to handle additional surrogate cases."

Because his original bill was getting bogged down in battles over details, Fitzpatrick decided to take a different tack. In March 1982, he introduced a different, streamlined bill, which paralleled the artificial insemination by donor (AID) laws in effect in many states. The bill said nothing about medical examinations of the surrogate or the natural father, nor did it address the contingencies of an abnormal child or the death of one or both of the couple. It set no limit on compensation. All the bill did was provide a procedure so that the man who used a surrogate would get legal custody of the child. Also, due to pressure on Fitzpatrick from adult AID children and adoptees who stressed the importance of a child learning his or her biological parent's name, the bill contained a controversial line allowing the child the right to obtain the surrogate's name unless she objected.

This second version of a surrogate bill progressed no further than its predecessor. It looked as if it would take some surrogate tragedy to propel the Michigan legislature into action on the issue. Then, such a tragedy happened.

In January 1983, a baby with microcephaly (a small head, indicating possible mental retardation) was born to surrogate mother Judy Stiver. Alexander Malahoff, the man who had provided sperm for her insemination and promised Stiver $10,000 to bear his child, decided he no longer wanted the child. He ordered the hospital to withhold treatment for the baby's staph infection. The hospital received a court order allowing it to treat the baby. The surrogate mother said that she felt no maternal bond to the child.

A few weeks later, blood tests showed that Malahoff was not the father of the child. Apparently Stiver had been told to abstain from intercourse with her husband for a month after the insemination but had not been told to abstain immediately before the procedure. She became pregnant by her husband, all the while thinking she was carrying Malahoff's child. Now she will not get paid her $10,000, she is keeping a child she did not want, and Malahoff is suing her for millions of dollars for not producing for him the baby he was promised.

Because of the Stiver-Malahoff controversy, Fitzpatrick realized that Michigan needed legislation that went beyond the bare bones approach in handling such situations. He wanted to make sure that the man contracting for a child could find out quickly whether he actually was the biological father and he wanted to ensure that a man who was the biological father could not reject a child with a defect.

"We don't all get the Gerber baby," observed Fitzpatrick, pointing out the importance of making the couple irrevocably responsible for the child. So Fitzpatrick introduced yet a third surrogate bill, taking a middle ground between the streamlined and detailed versions he had proposed earlier. The bill provides for medical, psychiatric, or psychological testing of the surrogate (but not of the man providing the semen) and requires the surrogate to adhere to medical instructions before and after the insemination and during pregnancy. The couple and surrogate must abide by their contract, but the law does not describe the provisions the contract should contain. Within twenty-four hours of the baby's birth, blood tests are performed to determine who the biological father is. The couple has legal responsibility for the child unless the husband proves he is not the father. Like the previous version, the law would allow the child to learn the surrogate's name when he or she reaches age eighteen if the surrogate agrees. A violation of the law by either side could lead to up to ninety days in jail and/or a fine of up to $10,000.

Fitzpatrick feels that this bill has a greater chance of passage than the previous two. "Previously, I could only speak of hypothetical problems that could possibly occur if everything didn't go smoothly in a surrogate situation," he comments. "With the recent Stiver-Malahoff case in Lansing, we can see what happens when the state has no rules or regulations. For weeks the baby was tossed back and forth like a football—with no one having responsibility. Had this legislation passed, the legal problem would not have existed."

Another Michigan legislator feels that the Stiver-Malahoff incident is evidence of why surrogate parenting should not exist at all. Representative Connie Binsfield, a former Michigan "Mother of the Year," drafted a law forbidding surrogate parenting altogether and subjecting those who violate the law to ninety days in prison, or a $10,000 fine, or both.

The four types of laws that have been proposed since 1981 in Michigan illustrate the varied approaches that can be taken to the regulation of surrogate motherhood. As with the artificial insemination laws that were enacted beginning in the mid-1960s, the laws that are ultimately passed could vary greatly from state to state. Unlike the AID laws, it is early enough in the legal process that you can make a difference in the law that your state passes. Contact your state legislator, band together with other infertile couples to present testimony at legislative hearings on surrogate motherhood, and let your voice be heard about the type of law you think your state should pass. Until there are clear laws on the books, there will continue to be unfair emotional and legal risks for the people who enter into surrogate arrangements. An editorial in the *Detroit Free Press* on January 25, 1983, said it best: "Surrogate parenting, no matter how we feel about the practice, is a phenomenon that isn't likely to go away. Properly regulated by specific and careful legislation, it could help to enrich lives. Unregulated or bound only by loose guidelines, it could become the spawning ground for countless tragedies."

• *SURROGATE MOTHERING—PAST AND FUTURE*

Although surrogate mothering has recently reached public attention, it is not a new phenomenon. Its use dates back to the Scriptures. When Sarah could not produce an heir for Abraham, she had him visit the tent of her young handmaiden Hagar.

Now, though, the matter is less personal. Since artificial insemination is used, the surrogate need not even be in the same state as the man who will father the child. Most surrogates today have no previous tie to the couples. Newspaper advertisements are used to match surrogates and couples. One ad in a California newspaper immediately drew responses from 160 potential surrogates.

The ranks of couples requesting surrogates are swelling as well. "We've got couples from all over the country as well as from Switzerland, Sweden, Spain, Germany, Italy, France, Lebanon, Argentina, Canada, Sri Lanka, and countries I'd never heard of before," says Karen Zena, coordinator of Surrogate Parenting Associates, Inc.

Why are an increasing number of couples expressing interest in using a surrogate? For one thing, the wait to adopt through normal agency channels is anywhere from three to seven years. And many couples delight in the fact that the baby will be related to them.

"It's special to me that the baby will have our heritage," declares Jane Kloner. "We knew that if there was any way possible to be at least somewhat biologically connected with the child, we'd do it."

9 ❦ Even Newer Conceptions—From Embryo Transfer to Embryo Freezing

The next decade promises to give rise to even more means of creating children for previously infertile couples. If science can make an artificial heart, the development of artificial tubes or an artificial uterus would seem to be well within the realm of possibility. Since infertility research is now beginning to focus on men's problems, we can expect to see new drugs developed to enhance men's sperm counts. For both sexes, intricate microsurgery and laser surgery will become even better developed to help repair damage to and defects of the reproductive organs.

In addition, many new means of achieving parenthood are possible through combinations of the New Conceptions described in this book. For example, a woman who can provide an egg but has no uterus could have her egg fertilized with her husband's sperm and then implanted in another woman. This combination of *in vitro* fertilization and a surrogate carrier could also be used by women who cannot carry a child due to a medical condition unrelated to fertility, such as high blood pressure.

It is now medically possible for a child to have five parents: an egg donor, a sperm donor, a woman who provides a uterus to gestate the child, and the couple who raises the child. Any combination of parenting could be used to meet an infertile couple's desire for a child. Among the possibilities are ovary transplants, egg donation, embryo transfer, artificial embryonation, embryo adoption, and *in vitro* or *in vivo* fertilization with a surrogate carrier. Further in the future are the possible use of embryo freezing, genetic screening *in vitro*—and perhaps even implanting an IVF embryo into the father to create a *male* pregnancy.

• *TRANSPLANTATION*

Some attempts have been made to treat infertility through transplantation of various reproductive organs from one person to another. A man born without testicles successfully achieved a pregnancy with his wife after he received a transplant of one testicle donated by his brother. In several instances, transplants of fallopian tubes have been undertaken, but there have been no reported births. In England, a British doctor had planned to help an infertile woman have children by doing an ovary transplant. The surgery was stopped, however, when British authorities informed the doctor that although his patient could then conceive and carry a child, any offspring that might result would be considered illegitimate. In the United States, however, the transplantation of ovaries would probably be likened to a kidney transplant and not be interfered with by authorities.

Even if ovary transplants were allowed, their value would be limited. A postmenopausal woman, for example, would not be able to conceive a child after receiving an ovary transplant from a younger woman. Research in rats has shown that when ovaries are transferred from young rats to old rats, the ovaries take on the pattern of the old rat. The ovary from an old rat, however, can be "turned on" by transfer to a young rat. This may mean that young infertile women without ovaries could receive an ovary transplant from an older woman (for example, one who is undergoing a hysterectomy) and have a chance at achieving a pregnancy.

Transplants of reproductive organs require major surgery and carry risks of rejection. Donors are difficult to recruit. For these reasons, researchers are exploring donation of female reproductive cells. Just as men now donate sperm, women are being asked to donate either unfertilized or fertilized eggs. Since women can successfully carry the offspring of other women, there is no rejection problem. It is easier to get donors of reproductive cells than of reproductive organs and, in some instances, the transfer can be done without surgery.

• *EGG DONATION*

Some women would be able to carry a child but are not able or do not want to provide the egg for the child. The woman may have been born without the ability to produce eggs, she may have prematurely entered menopause, she may have had her ovaries removed in an operation, her eggs may be unable to reach the site of potential fertilization due to adhesions on the ovaries or damage to the fallopian tubes, or perhaps she produces eggs but does not wish to conceive a child with her eggs because of the possibility of passing on a genetic defect.

For the woman who can provide the uterus for a child but not the egg, one answer in the future will be an egg donation. Already the use of the procedure is being explored by scientists in Italy. They call it TDO, the transfer of donor oocytes (eggs). Through a laparoscopy they extract an egg from the ovary of a woman donor. They use another laparoscopy to place the donated egg in the lower part of the fallopian tube of the recipient. The woman who receives the egg can then have sex with her husband or be artificially inseminated with his sperm in the hope that the sperm will fertilize the egg in her body and the pregnancy will develop normally.

All the scientific evidence indicates that it is possible to initiate pregnancy through the transfer of a donated egg. Such a procedure would be totally analogous to artificial insemination, in which donated sperm is used. Although it would be easier to find an egg donor than an ovary or fallopian tube donor, it still would be more difficult to find an egg donor than it is to find a sperm donor. While semen is usually collected in "masturbatoriums"—softly lit rooms filled with erotic magazines—collecting an egg necessitates surgery and thus presents greater danger.

Nevertheless, women in a number of situations may be willing to donate eggs. For example, women who are undergoing pelvic surgery for other reasons (such as a hysterectomy) may be willing to give up one or more eggs that the surgeon collects at that time. In addition they may be willing to take hormones such as clomiphene citrate or Pergonal in advance of their surgery so that they will be able to produce a number of eggs for donation. Several eggs could be transferred to one recipient or one or more eggs could be transferred to each of several recipients.

In the research studies undertaken when *in vitro* fertilization was first being explored, many eggs were obtained from women in just this manner—donation during surgery for other reasons. In addition, women currently undergoing *in vitro* fertilization may be willing to donate excess eggs since the drugs given to the IVF patients to stimulate ovulation sometimes produce too many eggs to be implanted safely after fertilization.

What would be the legal status of the child born after an egg donation? Since the law in the United States views the woman who gives birth to the child as its legal mother, the recipient would have no need to follow any particular procedure to assert a claim to the child she bears, even though it will not be genetically related to her. In addition, so long as the doctor obtained the informed consent of the egg donor and the recipient, there would seem to be no laws that would impede the physician from undertaking the egg donation procedure. Since the physician will be transferring an egg rather than an embryo, the fetal research laws and fetal experimentation laws will not apply to prohibit the transfer.

• *EMBRYO TRANSFER AND IVF WITH DONOR SPERM*

Researchers in Australia have made several creative uses of *in vitro* fertilization so that they can expand its application to a wider range of infertile couples. Some couples entering an *in vitro* program not only have a problem with female infertility (due, say, to blocked or absent tubes) but also have a problem with male infertility (due to an inability to produce sperm). For such a couple, traditional artificial insemination by donor is impossible, since the woman's eggs cannot travel down the fallopian tubes for fertil-

ization by the donor sperm. Standard *in vitro* fertilization is useless, too, since the woman's husband does not produce sperm that
can be used to fertilize his wife's egg *in vitro*. So Australian doctors use a combination of AID and IVF. They remove eggs from
the wife via laparoscopy, fertilize the egg *in vitro* with donor
sperm, and then implant the embryo in the wife.

At least twelve pregnancies have been achieved at the Queen
Victoria Medical Centre in Melbourne, Australia, using this technique. At the American Fertility Society meeting in April 1983,
Australian obstetrician John Leeton announced an additional exciting use of *in vitro* fertilization. With Dr. Alan Trounson, Dr.
Carl Wood and other colleagues at the Queen Victoria Medical
Centre, Leeton had fertilized a donated egg *in vitro* and transferred the resulting embryo to a recipient woman who became
pregnant.

The donor was a forty-two-year-old woman who had been trying
to conceive for four years. She underwent laparoscopy and five
eggs were removed for *in vitro* fertilization. She was advised that
not more than three embryos should be implanted in her because
of the risks associated with a multiple pregnancy.

"We only transfer back three embryos per patient," notes
Leeton. "We've already had four sets of twins and we now have a
woman pregnant with a set of triplets." When it is possible to remove more than three eggs, says Leeton, "the patient has to decide what to do with the excess."

"She has several choices," explains Leeton. "She can have them
left in the ovary, she can have them removed and frozen, or she
can donate them. This decision is made by the patient and her
husband. Our clinic has a waiting list of two years so there is
plenty of time for them to discuss it."

Most *in vitro* patients do not have excess eggs to spare. But
when Leeton's forty-two-year-old patient learned she had five
eggs, she requested that four be fertilized with her husband's
sperm and the other be donated.

The recipient in this case was a thirty-eight-year-old woman who
had been married for nineteen years, eighteen of which she had
been trying unsuccessfully to have a child. An evaluation of her

husband revealed that he had no sperm. Although she and her husband had one adopted child, they wanted another. She wanted the experience of pregnancy. She tried artificial insemination by donor, but after twenty-two attempts at insemination, she still had not conceived. So she entered the Queen Victoria Medical Centre program as a potential recipient.

When the forty-two-year-old *in vitro* patient decided to give up one of her eggs, the recipient was chosen because their menstrual cycles were synchronized to within twelve hours of each other. The donor egg was fertilized *in vitro* with sperm from an anonymous male (not the donor's husband or the recipient's husband, since he produced no sperm). The sperm was from a donor matched to the recipient's husband in terms of race, complexion, build, height, eye color, and blood group.

Three of the four eggs from the donor that had been fertilized by her husband's sperm were implanted in the donor. At about the same time, but in another facility, so that anonymity would be strictly guarded, the egg fertilized with donor sperm was implanted into the recipient woman.

In the Australian program, there are more potential recipients waiting for eggs than there are donors. Although the donors, participants in the *in vitro* program, receive hormones to regularize their cycle and stimulate the production of eggs, the recipients do not receive hormones. Instead, when a woman decides to donate an egg, the doctor chooses from the pool of potential recipients a woman whose cycle just naturally matches (or comes very close to) that of the donor.

"Synchronization is important," explains Leeton. "Each day we look for a matching between potential donors and potential recipients." The latter provide daily blood samples between day ten and day fourteen of their cycle and collect their urine every six hours at home on days eleven to fourteen, bringing it into the lab once a day for analysis. The doctors look for a recipient whose hormone picture matches that of the donor. Ovulation in the recipient must occur within twenty-four hours of that of the donor so that the recipient's uterus is at the correct stage for implantation of the embryo."

Although it may seem extraordinary that a woman would be able to carry an embryo that is not genetically related to her, it is medically possible for her to do so if her uterus is at just the right stage in the cycle for her to nourish the growing embryo. For the thirty-eight-year-old Australian woman, the embryo did implant itself nicely and begin to grow within her womb. Sadly, though, the woman miscarried in her tenth week.

The miscarriage does not indicate that this technique is destined not to work. Rather, the fetus was suffering from a genetic defect apparently not caused by the *in vitro* fertilization or the transfer to the recipient. Possibly the defect was due to the advanced age of the forty-two-year-old donor. Similar miscarriages occur with genetically defective fetuses that have been conceived naturally.

Leeton and his colleagues feel that embryo transfers of an egg fertilized *in vitro* offers new hope for infertile couples. A variation on the technique would be to fertilize the donor egg *in vitro* with sperm of the recipient's husband.

"This process could be used on women with absent ovaries or those carrying inheritable genetic disease, or those with a severe pelvic disease or abnormality preventing access to the ovaries for laparoscopic recovery, those whose ovaries don't respond to stimulation or those in whom *in vitro* fertilization has failed," elaborates Leeton. He also notes that the technique would be of value to women whose physical condition does not permit them to participate in the entire IVF process (for example, because of the dangers of anesthesia). Because the implantation of an embryo is not a surgical technique but rather is accomplished without anesthesia by gently expelling the embryo through a tube inserted into the uterus through the vagina, it offers less potential risk.

Addressing a group of infertility specialists from around the world at the American Fertility Society Annual Meeting in San Francisco in April 1983, Leeton acknowledged that he "recognized the legal and ethical problems" posed by the use of donated embryos. In the United States, it may take a challenge to the fetal research or fetal experimentation statutes of a particular state before such embryo transfers will be permissible. As to the status of the children, they will be the legal children of the women who bear them, even though they are not genetically related to the women. When donor sperm is used as well as a donated egg, however, the relationship of the woman's husband to the child will probably be governed by AID laws. Initially, when children were conceived by the use of donor sperm inseminated directly into the woman's vagina (that is, traditional AID) rather than by adding the donor's sperm to a petri dish holding the woman's egg, some courts held that the child had *no* legal father and that the wife committed adultery by undergoing donor insemination. The more recent court view is that it is not adultery and that the child is the legitimate child of both the woman who bears him and her consenting husband. In addition, twenty-four state legislatures have adopted laws to that effect. These laws would seem to make the husband the legal father, even if the donor insemination was performed in a petri dish rather than directly in the woman.

Leeton's concerns about the process go beyond the legalities, however. He worries about how the process can be designed to minimize destructive psychological effects on the parties. The ethics committee of Queen Victoria Medical Centre approved donated embryo transfer only if the donor and recipient remain anonymous, "thus preventing the possibility of interaction or argument between the genetic and rearing parents." Anonymity also helps avoid resentment about the recipient's pregnancy on the part of a donor who does not herself become pregnant. (None of the three embryos that had been implanted in the forty-two-year-old donor developed into a pregnancy, even though the one fertilized egg that she had donated did develop into a pregnancy in the recipient.)

"As more pregnancies occur the problem is less likely to arise," write the Australian doctors, "but in asking some women to donate their oocytes (eggs) it may be worthwhile pointing out the possibility that their original motivation to help someone else may increase their disappointment and lead to resentment should their own attempt fail."

Anonymity may be beneficial to the couple and the donor. However, warn the researchers, "This ignores the possible need of the child to identify the genetic parents as some adopted children have desired." Clearly, the many ramifications of donated embryo transfer will need to be worked out by society in the years to come.

• *ARTIFICIAL EMBRYONATION AND EMBRYO ADOPTION*

Because of the difficulties of transferring a donor egg or fertilizing it *in vitro* for embryo transfer, Randolph Seed, a physician, and his brother, Richard Seed, an embryologist, decided to experiment with a technique that relies more closely on nature. At their Reproduction and Fertility Clinic in Chicago, they are attempting to use volunteer women as human petri dishes.

Richard Seed explains the process: "Artificial embryonation is the transfer, four to five days after fertilization, of a human embryo from the uterus of a fertile donor to the uterus of an infertile recipient, who will then carry the embryo to term." In artificial embryonation (AE), a childless husband and wife pay a fee so that a fertile woman will be inseminated with the husband's sperm. If the egg is fertilized in the woman's body, an attempt is made four to five days after fertilization to flush out the embryo so that it can be implanted in the wife, as in *in vitro* fertilization.

In March 1983, Dr. John Buster, associate professor of obstetrics and gynecology at the University of California at Los Angeles, made the first known attempt at transferring a human embryo from one woman to another. In that case, a twenty-three-year-old woman was the recipient. Although she had previously conceived and had two unsuccessful pregnancies, she had been infertile for the previous three years due to infections and complication of surgery. Her thirty-five-year-old husband was fertile, with a high sperm count and good overall health.

A twenty-year-old fertile donor woman was matched as closely as possible on physical characteristics and blood groups and, most importantly, menstrual cycle timing, with the twenty-three-year-old. When monitoring of the fertile donor's menstrual cycle indicated that she was about to ovulate, she was artificially inseminated with sperm from the infertile woman's husband. A successful fertilization occurred *in vivo* (in the woman's body). Five days later, the fourteen-cell fertilized egg was withdrawn from her via a flexible plastic tube inserted in her uterus. The researchers examined the embryo under a microscope, photographed it, and then used another tube to insert the embryo in the recipient twenty-three-year-old. No surgery or anesthesia was used on either woman. According to Buster, neither woman experienced any discomfort.

Although that particular embryo did not successfully implant and grow in the recipient's uterus, the researchers continued their program and announced in July 1983 that two women had become pregnant through artificial embryonation.

In addition to offering artificial embryonation, the Seeds, Buster, and their colleagues hope to provide another form of *in vivo* fertilization followed by embryo transfer, known as embryo adoption. "The technology is the same as in artificial embryonation, but donor semen is used instead of the semen of the recipient's husband," explains Richard Seed. "In this case, the embryo has genes from neither of the 'adoptive' parents, even though the 'adoptive' mother will bear the child; thus the situation is analogous to the adoption of a child." Seed recalls how the idea came about. "It's amusing I didn't think of this myself," he says. "A patient called up and said he had been trying to adopt a child for five years, and asked, 'Why can't I adopt an embryo?' A few months later I called him back, and that started the whole thing."

Buster and the Seeds feel that transfers of embryos fertilized *in vivo* as part of AE or EA will someday eclipse the test-tube baby technique in popularity. After all, *in vivo* fertilization offers hope to more women than does traditional IVF since it can be used by women who have no ovaries, inaccessible ovaries, or who do not wish to pass on a genetic defect. In addition, it is potentially safer, since it requires no drugs, anesthesia, or surgery. Moreover, it is a less costly solution to female infertility than IVF or the use of a surrogate mother. *In vitro* fertilization costs $4,000 to $5,000 per attempt. Payment to a surrogate and the professionals in a surrogate mother program generally costs upwards of $20,000. With *in vivo* fertilization, the donor woman is paid around $250 for each menstrual cycle during which she is being monitored or inseminated, and the doctors can charge less than do those involved with IVF since the procedure is less involved.

The Seeds already have between two hundred and three hundred couples on their waiting list for AE and EA at their clinic. They seek women to serve as donors in much the same way as sperm banks seek men to provide semen; they advertise at medical schools. They also ask their infertile patients to try to recruit a friend to serve as a donor in the program. (To maintain anonymity and avoid potential emotional problems, the donor a couple brings to the program does not serve as their donor; instead, she is used by another couple.)

According to Richard Seed, the women they are seeking "have no genetic diseases, are between the ages of twenty-one and thirty-five, and have a sound emotional structure." They do not ask a psychologist or psychiatrist to interview the woman; rather, they do the donor screening themselves.

Seed believes that neither AE nor EA would involve any legal procedures. "We feel the child delivered to the previously infertile mother will be her child legally," he explained, "and her previously infertile husband will be the legal father, with no necessity for actual adoption proceedings." However, even though the status of the child may escape legal scrutiny, the actual *in vivo* fertilization and embryo transfer procedure might run afoul of existing state fetal research laws.

Louisiana law, for example, prohibits the "conduct on a human embryo or fetus *in utero*, of any experiment or study except to preserve the life or improve the health of said human embryo or fetus." In at least 17 other states, the statutes regulating fetal research might also prohibit the practice of embryo transfer. A greater number of fetal research statutes restrict this procedure than restrict *in vitro* fertilization. While *in vitro* fertilization is unaffected by statutes that prohibit fetal research in connection with an abortion, such statutes would prohibit AE and EA because the flushing technique generally falls within the definition of abortion. Moreover, the use of artificial insemination would bring the enterprise within the AID laws.

• IN VITRO *OR* IN VIVO *FERTILIZATION WITH A SURROGATE CARRIER*

The ability of a woman's egg fertilized *in vitro* or *in vivo* to be successfully transferred into and flourish in the uterus of a second woman gives rise to yet another possible scenario. What if a couple's infertility problem is due to the woman's inability to carry a child because of a problem with her uterus or a physical condition (such as severe diabetes or high blood pressure or a weak heart)? The couple could then explore either of two possibilities. The wife's egg could be fertilized with the husband's sperm *in vitro* and then implanted in a second woman, a surrogate carrier who agrees to carry the child for nine months, bear it, and then turn it back over to the couple. Or the couple could have intercourse, conceive naturally within the wife's body *(in vivo)* and then have the embryo removed five days later through the flushing technique and implanted in the surrogate carrier.

Infertility specialists see widespread potential for such techniques. "There are many woman, potentially fertile, who are advised against pregnancy, and the transfer of their embryos to a surrogate mother who would carry the fetus to full term would enable them to have their own children," writes Dr. Robert Edwards in the *Quarterly Review of Biology*. Richard Seed suggests that the technique would also be of particular value to women who can readily conceive but who miscarry.

The situation in which an embryo that is the genetic offspring of the couple is implanted in a surrogate carrier, gestated for nine months, then returned to the couple is radically different biologically from the already widespread surrogate mother situation. In the latter practice, the surrogate is artificially inseminated with the husband's sperm and thus provides half the genes as well as the womb for the child.

Even though the surrogate carrier is not genetically related to the child, she would probably still be considered to be the legal mother and her husband, if any, the legal father. The man who provided the sperm could try to bring a paternity action to prove by blood tests that he is the legal father. However, in no state is there a provision for a woman to bring a *maternity* action to prove that she is the biological mother of a child born to another woman. That is because the legal system, unprepared for the new reproductive methods, just assumes that the birth mother is the genetic mother.

If the man providing the sperm does successfully prove that he is the biological father, he could try to gain custody of the child. If his wife cannot prove she is the mother, she will have to adopt the child (even though it is genetically hers). This situation is legally (although not medically) analogous to the surrogate mother procedure and would have some of the same legal ramifications.

The going rate for a surrogate mother is anywhere from $5,000 to $20,000; surrogate carriers would probably charge about as much. There is evidence that more women would be willing to serve as surrogate carriers than as surrogate mothers. Detroit psychiatrist Philip Parker has found that some women would feel more comfortable renting their wombs for nine months than providing half the genes for the child as well.

Although some couples might be able to find a friend or relative to serve as a surrogate carrier, most would probably have to pay a woman to serve that role. This exchange of money may be viewed by some courts as baby-selling, thus running afoul of a number of state statutes, such as the antislavery laws, which prohibit the buying or selling of "people." The California penal code provides that giving or receiving money or anything of value in consideration of placing one person in the custody of another is punishable by a two- to four-year imprisonment. Yet the surrogate carrier has a stronger argument than does the surrogate mother that she is not selling a child. After all, she provides none of the genetic material, she just rents her womb.

The most extensive laws applicable to a surrogate mother arrangement are the adoption laws. In many states, payment in connection with an adoption (other than for limited, enumerated medical and legal fees) is forbidden. Some states make a special exception when one of the members of the adopting couple is the child's natural parent. To learn more about the rights and responsibilities you will have under the adoption laws when using a surrogate carrier, read the section in Chapter Eight on the laws governing surrogate motherhood.

Because of the legal uncertainties with respect to surrogate motherhood, legislatures in Alaska, California, Kansas, Michigan, South Carolina, and Tennessee are considering surrogate legislation. However, all of these laws deal with surrogate mothers who have been artificially inseminated (and thus provide an egg as well as a uterus for gestation). None of the legislatures has had the foresight to consider the surrogate carrier situation in which the couple's embryo is transferred to the surrogate after *in vitro* or *in vivo* fertilization. It is likely that additional laws governing surrogate carriers will be needed—perhaps laws that exempt people who use surrogate carriers from the adoption process on the grounds that a surrogate carrier is not giving up her child but giving back the genetic child of the couple.

• *FREEZING EMBRYOS*

Another option on the immediate horizon for infertile couples is the use of frozen embryos. Embryo freezing might offer several advantages to a couple. Hormone stimulation of a woman's ovaries during the IVF process may lead to the release of more than one egg. In most current IVF programs, if a number of eggs are removed and fertilized, all the ones that are developing are implanted in the woman. This has led to the birth of several pairs of twins. What if a large number of eggs were successfully fertilized—say, a half dozen or more? It might be dangerous to the mother or the embryos themselves to implant them all at the same time. With embryo freezing, the woman could bring to term some of the embryos and "save" the other embryos to be reimplanted at a later date. This approach may be the only way for a couple to space their children when, due to adhesions or other damage, a woman's ovaries are very hard to reach to perform the laparoscopy—such as when one ovary is blocked completely and the other offers only limited access. Because of extensive damage, a doctor may not be able to do a laparoscopy for the IVF procedure now and then do another one in a few years when the couple wants another child.

So, the physician may suggest that he or she stimulate the woman's ovaries with hormones, remove several eggs, fertilize them, implant one or two, and freeze the rest to be implanted at various stages when the couple is ready to expand their family. This eliminates the need for the second laparoscopy. A doctor may also suggest embryo freezing for a woman who is about to undergo radiation or other therapy that might damage her ovaries or possibly cause genetic mutation in the eggs. For years, sperm banks have offered frozen sperm. In this way, a man who is about to start taking drugs that might affect his fertility or who works in an environment that might be hazardous to sperm can have his healthy sperm frozen and later have a doctor use it to inseminate his wife.

Embryo freezing might also be employed in connection with embryo transfer or the use of a surrogate carrier. In that way, an embryo from one woman could be implanted, after freezing, into any other woman. When the implant takes place immediately after *in vitro* or *in vivo* fertilization, the recipient must have a menstrual cycle that is similar to that of the woman who produced the embryo. Freezing could keep the embryo at a certain stage until the recipient woman's cycle proceeded to the point where her uterus was prepared to accept an implantation.

With respect to embryo freezing, the Queen Victoria Medical Centre researchers in Australia—Alan Trounson, John Leeton, Carl Wood, and their colleagues—have once again taken the lead. Since they feel that it is medically appropriate to implant only three embryos after *in vitro* fertilization, they ask the woman whether she wants to freeze any excess embryos. In August 1982, they removed four eggs from a patient and successfully fertilized all four. They implanted three and, in compliance with the patient's wishes, froze the fourth. The woman became pregnant with one of the fresh embryos, but miscarried eight weeks later. In January 1983, the doctors thawed the fourth embryo and the woman achieved a successful pregnancy with that embryo.

In the United States, many of the *in vitro* fertilization clinics have the necessary equipment for embryo freezing. Although they are not undertaking research on embryo freezing at this point, they believe that the equipment is a necessary backup for their *in vitro* program.

"What if we can't locate the woman at the time her fertilized egg is ready for implantation?" asks one doctor. "What if she develops an infection from the laparoscopy and we are not able to implant immediately after fertilization? What if she's in a car accident on the way to the hospital for implantation? Even now, we need to have the capability to freeze the embryos since at least one of these scenarios has already materialized."

The use of frozen embryo banks, however, gives rise to myriad legal concerns. In its initial stages, it would be viewed as fetal experimentation in those states that define the term fetus to include embryos. In addition, the status of the frozen embryo will doubtless touch off endless debates. Who is responsible for a frozen embryo if the couple die? If a couple divorce and no longer want the embryo, can it be given to another infertile couple? Could a right-to-life group bring a legal action on behalf of an embryo claiming a right to be born—and perhaps even suggesting that one of its members would be willing to gestate the embryo? For inheritance purposes, should a frozen embryo be considered an extra child? All these questions, and many more, will be born of the embryo freezing technique.

• *GENETIC TESTING, GENETIC SURGERY, AND GENETIC TREATMENT*

In vitro fertilization and *in vivo* fertilization with embryo transfer put the embryo under scientific supervision at the earliest stages of its development. Some researchers have suggested that this could provide an opportunity for medical intervention to take place.

It might soon be possible to detect genetic diseases in an embryo while it is *in vitro* or before it is transferred to the second woman after *in vivo* fertilization and removal. In that way a woman will not have to undergo an amniocentesis five months into a pregnancy and then make the heart-wrenching decision about whether to abort a fetus that she might have already felt moving and kicking inside her. Instead, tests could be performed on one cell of the embryo to determine whether it had particular hereditary diseases or a chromosomal abnormality such as Down's syndrome. If the cell did have a defect, the couple might not wish to have the embryo reimplanted. This early testing would also give couples the opportunity to learn the sex of the embryo and perhaps forego implantation of an embryo they considered the wrong sex.

If a genetic defect were discovered at, say, the two-cell or four-cell stage, it might be possible to correct that defect by introducing genetic material into the embryo to compensate for the genes or gene products that are lacking. Such a genetic treatment becomes infinitely more complicated (if not impossible) in adult humans, who have trillions of cells rather than just a few and whose cells have already developed their specialized purposes.

The microsurgical techniques used to remove one cell of the embryo for testing could also be used to divide an embryo in half or quarters to create multiple, identical children. This is already done in cattle and sheep to increase the number of offspring from high-quality cows. Apparently, an embryo's dividing capabilities at its earliest stages are such that it can compensate for this intervention by undergoing extra divisions. Richard Seed foresees a day when "twinning" will be possible in humans: "That way we can bisect an embryo into two parts, implant one, raise that person until college age, see if it's all right, and then bring up the other one."

• *ANALOGOUS ANIMAL RESEARCH*

It will only be a short time before the techniques described in this chapter become widely available to infertile couples. Since they rely primarily on combinations of techniques discussed elsewhere in this book (such as artificial insemination, surrogate mothering, and *in vitro* fertilization), there are few scientific barriers to achieving these procedures. Moreover, researchers have already had widespread experience in using many of these procedures in animals.

As far back as 1890, researchers demonstrated that rabbit embryos could be flushed out of the genetic mothers, transferred to an unrelated surrogate carrier, and be born normally. This procedure is now a mainstay of the cattle industry. Although only about 250 commercial transfers were accomplished in 1972, now more than twenty thousand transfers are made each year. Cattle breeders use hormones to cause a prized cow to superovulate. She is then inseminated, either naturally by a bull or artificially with the sperm of a prized bull. (Bull sperm may sell from $2 to $60,000 a dose.)

Seven days later, a flexible catheter is introduced into her uterus and the fertilized eggs are flushed out, then implanted in other, less valuable cows. This allows high-quality cattle to produce many more offspring than they would in the normal manner. Since they do not carry their embryos to term, they can begin the process all over two months later. In this way, farmers use the top ten percent of their cattle to transfer offspring to the remaining ninety percent.

Embryo transfer has also been used to "upgrade" other species. Dr. R. F. Seamark, professor of obstetrics and gynecology at the University of Adelaide, Australia, reports, "We have transferred embryos from superior angora goats into wild goats." This allows the highly sought-after angora goats to have many more children than they themselves could carry to term and stops the wild goats from having their own scruffy offspring.

"Many experiments have been made on animals and successful embryo transplants after *in vivo* fertilization have been made in fourteen species," remarks Richard Seed. "Of the thousands of transplants done on cattle, there are no excess abnormalities. The second generation of these cattle are okay. And there have been no new abnormalities created."

Similarly, research with laboratory and domestic animals has found that transfer of an embryo fertilized *in vitro* to a genetically unrelated mother has not led to an increased number of abnormal offspring. Likewise, when mouse eggs are frozen, fertilized *in vitro,* and transferred to surrogate mothers, normal newborns have resulted.

Scientists still urge caution in the use of these techniques in humans, though. Dr. Richard Blandau, a professor at the University of Washington School of Medicine in Seattle, points out that the animal data must be put in perspective. Humans carry more genetic defects than do cattle and it may be difficult to analogize cattle defects to human ones. After all, asks Blandau, "Who would be concerned over any deficiency in creative ability in sheep?"

Nevertheless, the experience with artificial insemination and *in vitro* fertilization indicates that the human egg, sperm, and embryo are very resilient and there is no reason to expect that egg donation, AE, EA, embryo donation, or *in vitro* or *in vivo* fertilization with a surrogate carrier will give rise to any extra genetic difficulties.

Egg or embryo freezing, however, might create some risk. "There is no evidence that freezing itself is mutagenic," writes Dr. John D. Biggers of the Harvard Medical School in the *New England Journal of Medicine*. "However, it has been suggested that the cumulative effect of background radiation may increase the mutation rate, since no DNA repair will occur at the temperature of liquid nitrogen."

Short-term freezing, however, is unlikely to lead to increased genetic risk. If it becomes possible to do genetic screening on the embryo, testing for abnormalities of frozen embryos stored for long periods could be done before a decision is made whether or not to implant it.

• *MALE PREGNANCY*

The animal research also points the way toward a dazzling scientific coup that could raise myriad social, emotional, ethical and legal issues: male pregnancy. Dr. Cecil Jacobsen of George Washington University Medical School fertilized a chimpanzee egg *in vitro* with chimpanzee sperm, implanted it in the abdomen of a male chimpanzee, later delivering a healthy baby chimp through a Caesarean section. Australian researchers predict that the technique could be adapted to male humans, leaving open the possibility of surrogate fathers.

• *EMOTIONAL ASPECTS OF THE NEWER CONCEPTIONS*

The emotions of the couples using the techniques described in this chapter are much the same as with *in vitro* fertilization, artificial insemination by donor, and surrogate motherhood. To avoid the emotional minefields that could accompany a new reproductive technology, the couple must first come to terms with their infertility. When a third party is brought into the marriage relationship to aid in conception, great care must be taken so that the spouse who is being "replaced" by that third party does not feel left out. For example, if donor sperm is used to fertilize the wife's egg *in vitro,* an effort should be made to ensure that the husband participates in all other aspects of the procedure.

One especially difficult emotional aspect of using the techniques described in this chapter is their experimental status. Couples must be psychologically prepared for the high likelihood that the procedure will fail and they will not become parents. For some couples, the alternatives of trying a private adoption or remaining childless may be emotionally preferable to getting their hopes up one more time and having them dashed.

Before undertaking one of these procedures, couples should discuss freely their feelings about the technique and about the various potential outcomes. They should try to envision how they will feel if the process does not work and try to gauge how long they will keep trying if they do not initially achieve a pregnancy. They should discuss all possible scenarios that might occur even if at the moment they seem inconceivable. If they are using a surrogate carrier, they should explore how they will feel and what they will do if she decides to keep the child. If they are having an embryo frozen, they should determine what they will want done with the embryo if their marriage breaks up or one of them dies.

The couple should also take into consideration the viewpoint of friends, relatives, and society at large about the particular procedure they are using. This does not mean that they should forego a particular option just because, for example, their parents do not approve of their use of a surrogate carrier. Rather, the couple must decide how they will withstand the negative criticism and what might be done to make critics feel more comfortable with the idea.

• *THE FUTURE OF NEW CONCEPTIONS*

The New Conceptions are here to stay. As John F. Kennedy once said about nuclear physics, there is no way to return the genie to the bottle. Even if the new methods were banned in one country, research would be undertaken elsewhere.

The New Conceptions are important advances to help couples conquer infertility and, say some researchers, to help society protect itself from destruction.

"With the growing number of assaults to fertility," believes Dr. Robert Francoeur, professor of human sexuality and embryology at Fairleigh Dickinson University in Rutherford, New Jersey, "artificial insemination and embryo transfer could become a question of survival."

Biologist Bentley Glass, a professor emeritus at the State University of New York at Stony Brook and former president of the American Association for the Advancement of Science, sees another use for the new reproductive technologies. "Our only sensible civil defense against nuclear war is to build labs underground that are self-contained and preserve the reproductive cells of all the plants and animals necessary to reestablish life on this planet," he declares. In Glass's plan, human reproductive cells would be banked there, in a sort of modern-day version of Noah's ark.

But the application of the New Conceptions goes far beyond their ability to provide children to the childless or serve as a nuclear fallout repopulation plan. The new technologies could be applied to shape the way human beings develop by making improvements on nature through the choice of donor sperm and eggs or by rewriting the genetic code of an individual via genetic surgery.

"External human fertilization is an obvious symbol that we— frail, flappable, and fallible—are taking life into our own hands, including our humanity," states Clifford Grobstein in *From Chance to Purpose: An Appraisal of External Human Fertilization.*

Biologist and ethicist Leon Kass notes that the chain of human existence has traditionally been continued by a joining of the "pleasure of sex, the communication of love, and the desire for children." Those factors are not necessarily a part of the New Conceptions, however.

The possibility of procreation divorced from these basic human values is revolutionary. "The wrench is epic in human history," asserts Grobstein. "However cleverly biological consequences may be technically minimized, the translocation cannot fail to generate profound emotional, cultural, and social reverberations."

At this new crossroads in biology, University of Toronto philosophy professor Abbyann Lynch has posed the question for society most succinctly: "Ought man to apply technological skill to his own shaping?"

For some people, the answer is yes. Theologian Joseph Fletcher feels that the creation of our children should not be dependent on "the accidents of romance and genetic endowment, of sexual lottery." Biologist E.S.E. Hafez of Wayne State University is even more blunt: "We should breed people who produce good quality work and cut out the lazy types not interested in contributing to society. We already do this in race horses and dairy cows."

The late Nobel Prize winner Herman J. Muller had similar ideas: "Foster pregnancy, which is already possible, will become socially acceptable and even socially obligatory. It will seem wrong to breed children who mirror parents' peculiarities and weaknesses. In the future, children will be produced by the union of ovum and sperm, both derived from persons of proved worth, possibly long deceased, and who exemplify the ideals of the foster parents." Even beyond choosing donors of merit, genetic manipulation of the embryo could be used to produce "superior" children.

This view is a frightening one. Who is wise enough to decide what traits the human race should have? Even if people could reach a consensus on the optimal genetic endowment of the human race, would the breeding of humans for highly specific traits be biologically desirable?

A wide cross section of American religous leaders in June 1983 signed a resolution urging a ban on human genetic engineering. They favored gene therapy that would cure a given individual's defects but vehemently rejected engineering that would alter an egg, sperm, or embryo in a way that could be passed on to the next generation. According to the prestigious group, which included Roman Catholic bishops, heads of Protestant churches, Jewish leaders, the head of the Moral Majority, the president of the National Council of Churches, the presiding bishop of the Lutheran church, and the president of the Southern Baptist Convention, "engineering fundamental changes of human sex cells necessitates that decisions be made as to which genetic traits should be programmed into the human gene pool and which should be eliminated; and . . . no individual, group of individuals, or institutions can legitimately claim the right or authority to make such decisions on behalf of the rest of the species alive today or for future generations. . . ."

Abstractly, the idea of trying to create a "perfect" child is appealing. But the forced elimination of "genetic inferiority" would have deprived us of some of the world's greatest citizens—such as Dostoyevski, who was an epileptic, or even Abraham Lincoln, who had a congenital disease causing a number of "defects," such as abnormal-size fingers and toes.

Selective breeding could lead to social harm, such as a despotic leader trying to create a race of soldiers. It could lead to biological harm as well. Eliminating genetic variety would reduce human beings' ability to adapt to changes in the environment. Humans would be sentenced to the fate of the dodo and dinosaur, who became extinct when they could not adapt to a changing world.

"Since part of the strength of our gene pool consists in its very diversity, including defective genes, tampering with it might ultimately lead to extinction of the human race," warns Jeremy Rifkin, author of *Algeny,* a critique of genetic engineering. "It should be recalled that in the 1950s genetic modifications were made in wheat strains to create bumper crops of 'super wheat.' When a new strain of disease hit the fields, farmers found that their wheat was too delicate to resist. Within two years, virtually the entire crop was destroyed."

Also, by trying to create humans with a particular trait such as intelligence, society might lose out on other traits, such as cooperation or lovingness.

"Plants and animals are bred for one characteristic at a time," comments microbiology professor Bernard Strauss of the University of Chicago. "If you want a turkey with a lot of breast meat you can get it, but you might lose other traits." In breeding for intelligence or other specific traits in humans, it is not clear what valuable characteristics might get shortchanged.

The New Conceptions could change the notion of parenting and the nature of the human race. Making sure that this potential is used wisely is a task for all of us. As Nobel Prize winner Dr. James Watson has suggested, this is "a matter far too important to be left in the hands of the scientific and medical communities."

10 ❦ Parenting and the New Conceptions

"When I finally became pregnant after several years of trying," recalls Judy Calica, a clinical social worker and Resolve infertility counselor, "I felt like I was carrying an extremely fragile vessel inside of me. I was terrified that I might do something to lose the baby."

The infertile couple are used to disappointments. They have tried doing what comes naturally to most people and failed. They may have tried drugs or surgery to enhance their fertility with no results. Along their quest for pregnancy, their hopes have risen and been dashed dozens of times. Her period is a few days late, excitement rises, but no pregnancy follows. They read about a new treatment and start calling doctors, only to learn that it does not apply to them.

Then, the miracle occurs. Through *in vitro* fertilization, artificial insemination by donor, use of a surrogate, or some other new reproductive technology, a pregnancy occurs. The couple is joyful, but cautious. They wonder, is this just another of nature's cruel hoaxes?

A woman who becomes pregnant through *in vitro* fertilization knows that the time period immediately after the embryo is introduced into her body is a crucial one. She will rest quietly for the first few days to give the embryo a chance to lodge in the wall of the uterus. But this delicate, cautious approach to the start of the pregnancy may carry over to the months that follow. Even after the embryo is implanted and the fetus' development is safely under way, the IVF mother may still feel a greater need to limit her activities to protect her pregnancy than do women who get pregnant naturally.

The woman who becomes pregnant through artificial insemination by donor also feels that her pregnancy is different. Since she herself is fertile, she is less concerned than the IVF mother that she might lose the pregnancy. Rather, her concern focuses on the health of the child. Particularly if her doctor has not explained fully his or her method of donor selection, the woman may fret constantly through the pregnancy that the child may suffer from a defect transmitted from the sperm donor.

Although it is natural for any mother to be concerned about the health of her unborn child, the AID mother's fears about the process itself may exaggerate these concerns. Brenda, who was inseminated with sperm that had been frozen, worried for nine months that the freezing process itself had damaged the sperm and that she would give birth to an unhealthy child.

When a surrogate mother is used, couples are overcome with not only medical concerns but also the fear that the surrogate might try to keep the child.

"When I learn that my surrogate is pregnant," says Jane Kloner, "I may tell my family and some friends but I won't have a wholesale celebration. After nine years of infertility problems, I know that a pregnancy is still a long way from being able to hold a child in your arms."

In another couple using a surrogate, the husband is anxious about the possibility that the surrogate may try to keep the child. "My wife has been through so much trying to give me a child," he reflects, "I worry that she will be devastated if this method fails, too."

• THE BIRTH

Somehow, miraculously, the pregnancy passes. Finally, after all those years of waiting, a new member joins your family. Despite your longing for this child, his or her actual arrival may take some getting used to. When the surrogate hands you your baby, or when you visit the nursery to peek at your newborn IVF or AID child, your initial thought may be, "Who is this little stranger?"

Don't worry if you do not feel an immediate bond with the baby. Although you may think that the hesitation or distance you feel is due to the baby's unique conception, virtually all parents take a little while to develop a maternal or paternal feeling about the child. After all, parents may give a baby life, but once he enters the world, he is his own little person. A baby has his own temperament, his own interests—and the baby's personality takes a little getting used to.

"The job of raising any child is stressful," notes Resolve counselor Lynn Drew, "but a previously infertile couple may have no channel for letting off steam. They may feel that they have no right to complain about any aspect of child-rearing."

After years of saying that you would give your right arm to have a child, you may feel a little sheepish about complaining about washing diapers or getting up for 2:00 A.M. feedings. "Relatives may be impatient about listening to any gripes from previously infertile couples who finally have a child," observes Drew. It is important to air those concerns, however, so that they will not smolder and turn into resentment.

• *AVOIDING OVERPROTECTION*

For the most part, those who seek help with infertility have given careful thought to parenting. "They will be responsible parents," Patrick Steptoe told a conference of doctors, scientists, and ethicists, "probably much more so than many of the couples who have a high percentage of unplanned and unwanted pregnancies." But they may have to avoid overprotecting the child.

As the three of you grow into a family, the protective feelings you had during the pregnancy may continue. "I had ten miscarriages before I gave birth to Sylvia," relates one woman. "She's five now, but I'm afraid I might lose her, too. I worry that I may be overprotecting her, keeping her from friends so that she won't catch their colds."

Perhaps at the root of overprotection is the couple's fear that they will not be good parents unless they shelter and dote on their child. This can be stifling to the child, however, and may impede his or her ability to develop a sense of responsibility and independence. Instead, turn your concern for your child into extra encouragement and attempt to help your child develop his or her own interests and the ability to pursue those interests independently.

"The social couple who have invested so much in propagating may too heavily weigh their own needs and wishes on the child," warns Wayne State University sociologist Greer Litton Fox.

The lengthy quest you undertook to conceive a child should not be translated into unrealistic desires about what you expect from the child. The need to think of your child as just as normal as any other child was brought home humorously to Mary Harrison, author of *Infertility: A Guide for Couples.*

"How long did it take you to have me?" her young son asked.

"Five years," she replied.

"Oh," he said, "I just thought it was nine months."

• WHAT WILL THE CHILD BE LIKE?

Those of you embarking on raising a New Conceptions baby may wonder what that child will be like. Since the first test-tube babies and children of surrogate mothers are now just entering kindergarten, it will be years before we know how they compare intellectually, socially, physically, and psychologically to other children. Thus far, we do know that the health of these children is similar to that of children conceived in the usual manner. Since artificial insemination has been in use for a longer period of time, there has already been research on the development of AID children. The extensive literature on adoption also provides clues about what happens when children join a family in other than the old-fashioned manner.

Robert Edwards, who along with Patrick Steptoe "fathered" the test-tube baby technology, addressed the issue of the IVF child's development in an article in *The Quarterly Review of Biology.* "[T]here could be psychological or other problems in store for children conceived through fertilization *in vitro*," he wrote. "Most evidence would suggest an opposite conclusion: the children would give thanks to be alive, just as the rest of us do, for they would be the children of their own parents, born into a family where they are wanted for their own sake." He speculated that if publicity were avoided, "the children should grow and develop normally and be no more misfits than other children born today after some form of medical help."

If research in other areas holds true, test-tube babies and other New Conceptions children will fare even better than the bulk of children conceived normally. AID children garner higher scores on I.Q. tests than children from the general population. This is due to a number of factors common to other New Conceptions: the couple who use this means of parenting are generally fairly well-educated, middle- or upper-class people who are attentive to encouraging their children's mental and physical development.

Studies of how adoptive children fare may also provide some understanding of children born through artificial insemination by donor, surrogate motherhood, egg donation, embryo transfer, artificial embryonation, or embryo adoption. There are now five million adoptees in the United States; extensive research has shown that adopted children compare favorably with other children in terms of their mental health and adjustment. English researchers who conducted a follow-up study of all children born during a week in 1958 found that adopted children did equally well or better than other groups of children on measures of ability and attainment. Other studies show the profound influence of the couple who raise the child. Children are more similar to their adoptive parents than to their biological parents in their attitudes, intelligence, and moral standards.

When a couple rely on any type of donor or surrogate to help them attain a pregnancy, the infertile spouse wonders whether he or she will have an impact on the personality of the child. "I use an example to show people how great the influence of a non-biological parent is," says social worker Beth Bridgman, founder of the Hagar Institute, a surrogate mother program in Topeka, Kansas. "My mother died when I was two and I was raised by my stepmother. I have my stepmother's manner of speech, gestures. I even look like her. You can allow yourself the thrill of seeing yourself reproduced in your child, even if you are not biologically related." This is especially true with the New Conceptions, since an attempt is made to match the physical characteristics of the donor or surrogate to that of the infertile spouse.

• *PARENTAL POINTERS*

On the basis of adoption research, there is some advice about parenting that can be given to people who become parents via the new reproductive technologies. The adoptive parents who are most likely to rear well-adjusted children are those who view themselves as the real parents and minimize the role of the biological parents. Similarly, a couple who use a surrogate to achieve a pregnancy should view the stand-in mother as carrying *their* child. They likewise should think of the sperm donor or embryo donor as providing the biological building blocks for their own child, not as another "parent."

Many couples wonder whether a child born through artificial insemination, surrogate mothering, egg donation, artificial embryonation, or embryo adoption will be a constant reminder to the sterile spouse of his or her deficiency. Much of the original psychiatric literature in this area stressed these pitfalls. More recently, however, studies have shown that of the infertile people who rely on a third-party donor to help their spouses become parents, nearly three quarters feel that the children are as much their own as if they had been a genetic parent.

One point that has been especially tricky for adoptive parents is discipline. Some adoptive parents hold back, feeling they do not have the right to be stern with children created by someone else. Research on AID children found that fathers are reluctant to discipline the child. Setting limits on a child's behavior is an important means of showing that you care about that child and demonstrating that you are the real parent, whether or not you have a biological link.

Understanding your expectations for your child is necessary as well. If you worry that your child may turn out badly because of some unknown trait passed on by the surrogate, egg donor, or sperm donor, you may unwittingly convey that negative attitude to the child.

"Parents who fear the worst from their children often get it," explains New York psychologist Jacqueline Hornor Plumez in *Successful Adoption.* "Research shows that adoptive parents who are concerned about heredity or 'sexual promiscuity' of birth parents will tend to have problems with their children."

If a child is aware of his or her unique origins and has questions about how he or she entered the world, be sure not to brush off those concerns. The good communication you establish can carry over to other topics and other aspects of the parent-child relationship. Just as a couple's relationship is strengthened when they speak openly to each other about their feelings about infertility, a family relationship can be strengthened by the manner in which you answer your child's questions about his or her origins.

• *WHAT TO TELL YOUR CHILD ABOUT THE NEW CONCEPTIONS*

If your child begins life in a petri dish, you probably will want to tell him or her about this unusual beginning. By the time the child reaches the age of understanding, there will be hundreds (or even thousands) of other children born through *in vitro* fertilization, so the news should not make him or her feel strange.

"I'll tell our child about the conception and how much we wanted the baby," says IVF mother Ellen Casey, who gave birth to Elizabeth on August 3, 1983. "I'd even like to take her to Houston to visit the clinic and see where life began." The Caseys have a unique scrapbook to share with their child. "I have pictures of our baby since she was an egg on the surface of my ovary," boasts Ellen.

Most couples who are using surrogate mothers also intend to tell the child. Frankly, it would be difficult to keep the matter confidential. It will be obvious to family and friends that the wife is not the mother, since she will not be pregnant. The assumption will be that the child is adopted, so the issue is whether you should tell people (and most importantly, the child) that the husband is actually the genetic father. "We've decided that our child has the right to know about his special heritage," state one couple who are using a surrogate. They have even made tapes of television shows dealing with surrogate mothers to help them explain the situation to the child.

When a couple use artificial insemination by donor, however, the choice becomes more complicated. The same tough choice is faced by a couple who achieve pregnancy after egg donation, embryo transfer, artificial embryonation, or embryo adoption.

To tell or not to tell. That is a momentous decision that colors the couple's relationship with all others in their world. Since the pregnancy is carried by the wife, even though the sperm, egg, or embryo may be from a donor, people assume that the wife's obvious pregnancy was conceived by her and her husband. What are the costs or benefits of telling the truth to parents, friends, coworkers—and the children themselves?

Most doctors advise couples to maintain absolute secrecy. "If you have told anyone that your husband is sterile," one AID doctor warns patients, "go back and tell them a cure has been found so then they won't know that the child is not his."

In other countries, there is less agreement that secrecy is always appropriate. "In France, infertility seems to be less taboo," reports Simone Novaes, a sociologist who researches artificial insemination for France's National Center for Scientific Research. "Social paternity [as opposed to biological paternity] is more accepted in France than in the United States. There is more discussion as to whether the child should be told."

According to researchers Christine Manuel, Marie Chevret, and Jean-Claude Czyba, who work with couples at one of the main artificial insemination centers in France, 72 percent of the couples decided to maintain total secrecy and not tell anyone about the AID. Some couples, especially those who live in rural areas or are in the lower income levels, keep quiet because they feel that public sentiment is against AID.

As the public begins to understand the AID process and to realize how extensive it is (with upwards of ten thousand AID children being born yearly in the United States), couples may feel less need to maintain secrecy. Barbara Menning, founder of Resolve, predicts a trend in the direction of disclosure. Betty Orlandino tells the AID couples who are her clients at Human Relations Counseling that they should at least consider the possibility of telling the child.

Disclosure should not be made lightly. Unlike adoption or surrogate motherhood, where the mother-to-be is obviously not pregnant, there is nothing visible to distinguish the couple who use other New Conceptions from any other couple expecting a child. It *is* possible to maintain secrecy for a lifetime. If the husband will be more likely to feel the child is *his* child if the AID is not openly discussed, or the wife who uses an egg donor will feel a closer bond if the donor is not mentioned, then it is probably to the psychological benefit of the couple and child not to reveal the input of the third and fourth parties to the pregnancy.

A group of Dutch doctors performs artificial inseminations with donor sperm in the evening, after their clinic has closed, so that only the physician and the couple are present. Many American infertility specialists who perform AID let the obstetrician to whom they refer the couple assume the pregnancy was achieved naturally. The same could be done with egg or embryo donation so that the couple would be able to maintain secrecy if they wish.

"I advise my clients not to tell their AID children about their origins," comments infertility counselor Dr. Andrea Shrednick of New York. "I don't equate that to hiding something. My husband and I have two children born naturally and we haven't shared with them the details of their conceptions."

Before you decide to tell *anyone* about the use of a donor, you and your husband must decide whether you will tell the child. Once you have informed even a single individual—your mother, your best friend, your brother—you will have lost control of the information. There will now be a chance that your confidante will someday slip up and let the child know. The question of whether the child should be told should be faced early.

There is no easy answer. The child's best interest should be the guide. Keeping confidentiality might allow the child to grow up without the complications adopted children face of identity crises and fantasies of how much more wonderful his or her "real" father must be than his or her social one. Disclosure may be preferable, though, if it would alleviate the child's worries or provide a more serene home atmosphere. If AID was chosen because the husband had a genetic disease, knowledge that he or she was conceived by AID can be comforting to the child. One seventeen-year-old boy was upset about his own future when he found out that his father was dying of a genetic illness. When he learned that he had been conceived through AID and thus would not inherit the disease, he was grateful for his father's foresight. If secrecy would cause tension between you and your spouse, it might be wiser to be open with the child than have him or her grow up subconsciously feeling responsible for the rift between his or her parents.

"Despite the protective function of secrecy," wrote Manuel, Chevret, and Czyba in a report of their study of AID couples, "its preservation may have a high psychological price: if the very deep and legitimate need to communicate and share has to be defended against constantly, the secret itself may become a toxic and burdensome factor."

"When you start having secrets," observes psychologist Aphrodite Clamar, "it dictates the direction of your life. Keeping the secret can become much more important than the effect of keeping the secret."

Sadly, if the couple is not comfortable with the secret, they may break it to the child hastily and under unpleasant circumstances. In Annette Baran's study of AID children, she found that "the few children that were told anything were told in a punitive way or a frightened way." In one case, the husband, angry at his wife, told the child, "I'm not really your father."

In another case, the couple divorced and the husband's new lover taunted the wife that she knew about the AID. "The wife was afraid the girlfriend would tell the children, so she told them quickly out of fear," recalls Baran.

The couple have to work out what is most comfortable for them. They should discuss their concerns with each other. Some women are angered by secrecy, feeling they must constantly be covering up for their husbands. Similarly, some husbands would prefer disclosure because they feel reminded of their infertility every time someone congratulates them on becoming a father. A conversation with your spouse about disclosure should always come back to the crucial issues: What can we live with? What would be best for the child?

"The best time to tell is probably the mid to late teen years, when the child is already feeling stable about who he is," advises Orlandino. "When the child is just entering adolescence is probably not a good time because he generally will already be questioning who he is and what he is."

Children take their cues from their parents and can handle the news of their unique conception if their parents are comfortable with it. "In France, there was a radio program on secrecy in AID," says Novaes. "A thirteen-year-old boy called in and said, 'I don't know what the big deal is. I'm an AID child and I was told by my father.'"

"Children are less upset by apparently unpalatable facts than by any form of deception," explains Baran.

In a poignant article in *The New York Times Magazine,* Lillian Atallah discussed her feelings about being told at age nineteen that she was an AID child. "Knowing about my AID origin did nothing to alter my feelings for my family," she wrote. "Instead, I felt grateful for the trouble they had taken to give me life. And they had given me such a strong set of roots, a rich and colorful cultural heritage, a sense of being loved. With their adventure in biology, my parents had opened up the fairly rigid culture they had brought with them to this country. The secret knowledge of my 'differentness' and my sister's may have helped our parents accept . . . the few deviations from their norms that we argued for."

• *WHAT CAN THE CHILD LEARN ABOUT THE BIOLOGICAL PARENT?*

Some children who learn they were conceived with the help of a sperm donor, surrogate, egg donor, or embryo donor may want to learn that person's identity. Judging by the experience of adopted children, however, very few New Conceptions children will actually seek out information about their biological parents. In Scotland, although adult adoptees have a legal right to their original birth certificate, each year only 1.5 adoptees per 1,000 request the document.

Psychologist Howard Adelman predicts that the children born through the new reproductive technologies will be even less likely than adoptees to search for biological parents. "One of the forces in an adopted child's search for parents is the feeling that he or she has no roots, that he or she is being raised by two strangers," explains Adelman. "In the surrogate situation, the natural father is raising the child so he or she does have a feeling of roots." Similarly, with AID, the natural mother is raising the child, and with embryo transfer, the woman who has carried the pregnancy and given birth to the child is the one rearing him or her.

It is difficult to predict how many children born through the techniques discussed in this book will try to take legal action to trace biological links. It will be years before the children of surrogates, for example, reach adolescence and wonder about their identities. However, many thousands of people born through AID are already reaching adulthood. Scrutinizing what they do during the next few years will help predict the type of search for roots other New Conceptions children will make.

At age 31, Suzanne Rubin learned that the man she had called "Daddy" all those years was not her biological father. In 1948, her mother had undergone artificial insemination with sperm that she had been told was donated by a Los Angeles medical student. When Rubin learned the news, she felt betrayed—as if her entire life had been some sort of fiction. Determined to find her biological father, Rubin obtained the records of several hundred medical students enrolled in Los Angeles at the time. She is comparing the records and the students' pictures with the information her parents were given about the donor. For medical reasons and for her own peace of mind, she refuses to be detoured on the quest to find her biological father, the sperm donor. "I will either find him or I will find his grave," she says.

"AID children may begin to file lawsuits to learn the identity of their biological fathers, the donors of semen for AID," declares Jeffrey M. Shaman, a professor at DePaul University College of Law in Chicago. Already, legislator Richard Fitzpatrick reports that young adults who had been conceived via AID are lobbying the Michigan legislature to pass a law allowing them to learn the donors' identities.

"Should an AID child have the right to learn the natural father's identity?" asks Shaman. "There are two considerations that are contrary to each other. The child may have a great curiosity and psychological need to find out about his biological identity, and perhaps even a medical need. Yet it seems unfair to force the donor to take on the emotional obligations of parenthood when these were not his expectations. If courts begin to hold donors to an obligation of child support as well, it would ruin artificial insemination. No one would be willing to donate."

AID children searching for their donor fathers may follow the lead of some adopted children and take their quests to the courts. There is no constitutional right for an adoptee to see his or her adoption records, but some courts have allowed access to records in special circumstances—for example, when the child has a proven medical or psychological need.

Most states will allow adoptees to see their records only if they can prove they have some "good cause," but states differ in what they consider to be a good cause. Courts in the District of Columbia have given adoptees access if they have shown that there was a compelling need or that it would enhance their psychological welfare. One woman met that requirement by asserting that she needed to see her records to resolve her questions about her identity, to love and help her biological family, to learn her biological family's medical history to protect her children against hereditary diseases, and to ensure her children's rights to know their biological relatives. New York and Illinois courts have been more guarded, saying that the attainment of adulthood or curiosity about ancestors is not "good cause."

Even if AID children do win the right to see records of the insemination, the victory is apt to be disappointing. The majority of doctors do not keep records. In the eleven states that require insemination records to be filed with a state agency (Colorado, Connecticut, Kansas, Minnesota, Montana, Nevada, Oklahoma, Oregon, Washington, Wisconsin, and Wyoming), the records may be opened for "good cause." But there is no requirement that the donor's name be included in the record. Because every step of the adoption procedure is regulated by the state, adoption records are more detailed than those involving AID.

If a child of a surrogate files a lawsuit to gain access to information about his or her biological mother, the same requirement of "good cause" will apply. Since the adoption of a child of a surrogate is not done by a public agency, however, there may be little information in the record about the mother's background or medical history. The record may contain her real name, but the judge will probably be very reluctant to divulge that to the child.

Since medical research is discovering more and more links between genetics and the quality of a person's life and health, genetic counseling will be an increasingly important medical tool. Much of genetic counseling is based on the family health history, and a child born through one of the new reproductive technologies will not be able to participate in counseling if he does not know the medical background of his biological father or mother and other blood relatives. In the future, it may be necessary to enact laws to require that doctors keep such records and make them available to such children.

Already, some practitioners and sperm banks, notably Idant in New York, have extended donor family histories on file. The surrogate mother contract developed by attorneys William Handel and Bernard Sherwyn requires the surrogate to furnish them with any changes of address she makes for eighteen years after the child's birth, so that they will be able to contact her for medical and other information. Laws allowing a New Conceptions child to learn about the medical history of the biological parent but keeping confidential his or her identity would strike the delicate balance between the donor's or surrogate's right to privacy and the child's right to know.

• *HOW SHOULD YOU REACT TO THE SEARCH?*

In the past, many adoptive parents have been traumatized when their children sought out their biological parents. Searching for roots does not mean that the child does not love you or wants to live with the biological parent. Often, curiosity about the biological parent is a natural step in a child's development of his or her own identity.

Many adopted children have fantasies about their natural parents. Rock singer Deborah Harry, the lead singer of Blondie, was convinced that Marilyn Monroe was her natural mother. When one girl learned that she had been adopted in Washington, D.C., she looked back to see who was the president at that time. She was convinced that her natural parents were Dwight Eisenhower and one of his female staff members.

According to psychologist Dr. Zellig Bach, all children, no matter how they came into the world, tend to mythologize their parents. Children think their parents are the smartest, best-looking, most wonderful people in the world. For children to develop self-confidence and an individual identity, explains Bach, they must demythologize their parents and see them in a realistic light. Those children who know they have a biological parent somewhere yet know nothing about that parent may have trouble overcoming the fantasy.

If your child searches for the sperm donor or surrogate or other biological parent, don't let it hamper your relationship with the child. You may be angry at first. You will think it is unfair that this distant biological parent may reappear on the scene after you have done all the work of parenting. Where was the surrogate when you were changing diapers? Where was the egg donor when you stayed days on end at the hospital with a sick child? Where was the sperm donor when you gave up your vacation money to pay the child's tuition for another year?

Your bitterness about your child's search will not deter it. Rather, it will just make him or her feel guilty about the process. It may put the child in the position of feeling he or she has to choose between you and finding identity and peace of mind.

When children search for biological parents it is no reflection on the couple who reared them. They are not trying to replace that couple with a fantasy parent. Rather, they are trying to learn more about *themselves*. A large-scale study of adopted children by Arthur Sorosky, Annette Baran and Ruben Pannor found that "one of the striking aftereffects of reunions (between adoptees and birth parents) was the enhancement of the relationship between adoptees and their adoptive parents."

• WHAT RELATIONSHIP SHOULD YOU HAVE WITH THE BIOLOGICAL PARENT?

In some instances, the biological parent is more than the subject of your child's fantasy or a brief reunion. That person may play a concrete ongoing role in your life. A number of couples, for example, have used a friend or relative as a surrogate.

If you do choose a known individual to help you, you must work out carefully the type of relationship that person will have with the child. Decide in advance whether or when the child will be told of the special relationship and under what circumstances the person will be able to spend time with the child. In one of the more unusual—but apparently harmonious—arrangements, a surrogate is living with the couple for whom she bore two children. The wife is her best friend.

Even in situations where a previously unknown individual takes a role in a pregnancy, some couples agree to give that person access to the child. "I may be unusual," concedes Jane Kloner, who is contracting with a surrogate, "but I would not mind if the surrogate wanted visiting privileges."

Many couples and surrogates have agreed that if the child wishes to meet the surrogate, he or she will be allowed to. Even some sperm donors have said they will not discourage contact from their AID children. "I guess we can all use another relationship," says one donor.

Many surrogates and donors prefer not to have continuing contact with the couple, however. One surrogate who gets letters from the infertile woman who adopted the child says she would rather not have these painful reminders of the biological child she gave up. Another surrogate did not want to meet the couple whose child she was carrying. Inadvertently, she learned that they lived two blocks away and were friends of one of her neighbors. Although the surrogate liked her home, she moved away to avoid looking outside in the summer and seeing the child she had given up.

• THE EXPANDED FAMILY

If contact with the biological parent is initiated or maintained, what might be the effect on society of this expanded family? Some opponents of the New Conceptions argue that the evolving reproductive technologies could lead to the destruction of the family as we know it. Sociologist Greer Litton Fox disagrees. She feels that the new reproductive technologies may lead to intense social awkwardness and a rethinking of relationships, since we do not even have a name to describe the relationship between the genetic father and the surrogate or the donated embryo and the birth mother. However, she points out, "Families have shown themselves to be as flexible in the past."

"I do not believe that society needs to maintain an unbending family structure for its survival," declares psychiatrist Philip Parker. "Society should give the greatest flexibility and choice to its members and allow them to adjust their own lifestyle and family arrangements to suit their own wants and needs."

Modern medicine, the law, public opinion, and religious teachings all shape the role that the New Conceptions will have on society. But it is you, the mother and father of this brave new baby, who will translate a scientific and social advance into a loving and joyful family.

❦ APPENDIX A

Glossary of Trade Names

The following is a list of trade names, including registered trademarks, of the drugs mentioned in this book.

Azulfidine: Pharmacia Laboratories
    Division of Pharmacia, Inc.
    800 Centennial Avenue
    Piscataway, NJ 08854

Clomid: Merrell Dow Pharmaceuticals, Inc.
    Subsidiary of the Dow Chemical Company
    Cincinnati, Ohio 45215

Danocrine: Winthrop Laboratories
    90 Park Avenue
    New York, NY 10016

Dimetane Tablets & Elixir: A. H. Robins Company
    Pharmaceutical Division
    1407 Cummings Drive
    Richmond, VA 23220

Furadantin: Norwich Eaton Pharmaceuticals, Inc.
    13-27 Eaton Avenue
    Norwich, NY 13815

Imuran: Burroughs Wellcome Co.
    3030 Cornwallis Road
    Research Triangle Park, NC 27709

Macrodantin: Norwich Eaton Pharmaceuticals, Inc.
    13-27 Eaton Avenue
    Norwich, NY 13815

Ornade Spansule Capsules: Smith, Kline, & French
    Division of SmithKline Beckman Corporation
    1500 Spring Garden St.
    P. O. Box 7924
    Philadelphia, PA 19101

Parlodel: Sandoz Pharmaceuticals
A Division of Sandoz, Inc.
Route 10
East Hanover, NJ 07936

Pergonal: Serono Laboratories, Inc.
280 Pond Street
Randolph, MA 02368

Robitussin: A. H. Robins Company
Pharmaceutical Division
1407 Cummings Drive
Richmond, VA 23220

Serophene: Serono Laboratories, Inc.
280 Pond Street
Randolph, MA 02368

Tagamet: Smith, Kline & French Laboratories
Division of SmithKline Beckman Corporation
P.O. Box 7929
Philadelphia, PA 19101

Valium: Roche Products, Inc.
Manati, Puerto Rico 00701

APPENDIX B
Glossary

Adhesion: an abnormal attachment of adjacent membranes by fibrous connective tissue.

Adrenal glands: two glands near the kidneys that produce hormones, including some sexual hormones.

Agglutination of sperm: the clumping together of sperm.

Amniocentesis: procedure in which a small amount of amniotic fluid is removed from the uterus of a pregnant woman to determine whether the fetus suffers from particular genetic or chromosomal defects.

Antibody: substance that fights or otherwise interacts with a foreign substance in the body.

Artificial embryonation: process by which artificial insemination of a woman results in an embryo that is flushed out five days after conception and implanted in a second woman, the wife of the man who donated the sperm.

Artificial insemination by donor (AID): the placement of donor semen into a woman's reproductive tract for purposes of conception.

Artificial insemination by husband (AIH): the placement of a husband's semen into the wife's reproductive tract for purposes of conception.

Aspermia: the absence of sperm and semen.

Azoospermia: the absence of sperm in the semen.

Basal body temperature (BBT): the woman's temperature upon awakening in the morning, before any activity.

Bicornuate uterus: congenital malformation of the uterus in which the upper part is divided into two hornlike projections.

Bilateral tubal exclusion: experimental sterilization procedure for women, in which silicone rubber plugs are inserted in the fallopian tubes.

Caesarean section: delivery of a baby via surgical incisions in the mother's abdomen and uterus.

Cannula: hollow tube.

Cautery: sealing tissues together with heat.

Cervix: the opening of the uterus into the vagina.

Chromosome: rod-shaped bodies in a cell's nucleus which carry the genes that convey hereditary characteristics.

Cryobank: place where frozen sperm is stored.

Conception: the fertilization of an egg by sperm.

Congenital defect: a characteristic or abnormality present at birth resulting from a genetic or chromosomal defect or acquired during prenatal development.

Corpus luteum: the special gland which forms in the ovary at the point where the egg is released and which produces the hormone progesterone in the second half of the normal menstrual cycle.

Cryptorchidism: undescended testicles.

Dominant genetic defect: abnormality which manifests itself when a single gene in a gene pair is defective.

Ectopic pregnancy: a pregnancy that implants anywhere but in the uterus, often used to refer to implantation in the fallopian tubes.

Egg donation: surgical removal of an egg from one woman for deposit into the fallopian tube or uterus of another woman.

Embryo: the conceptus up to the end of the second month of a pregnancy.

Embryo adoption: process by which artificial insemination of a woman with donor sperm results in an embryo that is implanted in a second woman.

Embryo transfer: the introduction of an embryo into a woman's uterus after *in vitro* or *in vivo* fertilization.

Ejaculation: the male orgasm at which time seminal fluid containing sperm is discharged from the penis.

Endocrine system: system of glands including the thymus, pituitary, thyroid, adrenals, testicles or ovaries.

Endocrinologist: a doctor specializing in diseases of the endocrine glands.

Endometriosis: a presence of pieces of uterine lining (the endometrium) in abnormal locations, such as on the fallopian tubes, ovaries, and abdominal cavity.

Endometrial biopsy: extraction of a small piece of tissue from the uterus for examination.

Endometrium: the lining of the uterus.

Epididymis: long organ attached to each testicle where sperm collect on their way to the vas deferens.

Estrogen: a female hormone, produced mainly in the ovaries from puberty until menopause.

Eugenics: attempt to improve the human species through the control of hereditary factors in procreation. Positive eugenics entails encouraging procreation among those with desirable genes. Negative eugenics entails discouraging procreation among those with undesirable genes.

Fallopian tubes: a pair of narrow tubes that provide passage of the egg from the ovary to the uterus.

Fertilization: the penetration of an egg by a sperm.

Fetus: conceptus in the womb from the end of the second month of pregnancy until birth.

Follicle: egg sac in the ovary.

Follicular stimulating hormone (FSH): a hormone produced in the pituitary that stimulates the ovary to ripen a follicle or follicles for ovulation.

Gamete: the reproductive cells, known as the sperm in the man and the egg (ovum or oocyte) in the woman.

Genes: substances that convey hereditary characteristics, consisting primarily of DNA and proteins and occurring at specific points on chromosomes.

Gland: a hormone-producing organ.

Gonadotropin: substance capable of stimulating the testicles or ovaries.

Gynecologist: a physician who specializes in diseases of the female reproductive system.

HCG or human chorionic gonadotropin: hormone extracted from the urine of pregnant women that can be injected to stimulate gonads, ovaries, or testicles.

HMG or human menopausal gonadotropin: hormone extracted from the urine of postmenopausal women that can be injected to stimulate the gonads, ovaries, or testicles.

Hamster test: test of a man's sperm's ability to penetrate a hamster egg, thought to be evidence of the sperm's general penetrating ability.

Hormone: a substance produced by an endocrine gland and carried by a bodily fluid to another organ or tissue where it has a particular effect.

Human leukocyte antigens (HLAs): certain proteins found on the surface of human cells.

Hypothalamus: the region of the brain that controls the action of the pituitary.

Hysterectomy: surgical removal of the uterus.

Hysterosalpingogram: an X-ray study in which dye is injected into the uterus to show the outline of the uterus and the degree of openness (patency) of the fallopian tubes.

Immunologic response: the presence of sperm antibodies in the woman or man making the sperm clump together, thus reducing their fertilizing ability.

Implantation: the embedding of the embryo (fertilized egg) in the lining of the uterus.

Impotence: the inability to achieve or maintain an erection of the penis.

In vitro **fertilization:** the process by which an egg is surgically removed from a woman, fertilized in a petri dish with a man's sperm and the resultant embryo implanted in the woman's uterus.

In vivo **fertilization:** the fertilization of an egg by a sperm within the woman's body. In normal pregnancy, the woman in whom the egg is fertilized carries the pregnancy to term. In artificial embryonation or embryo adoption, the embryo is transferred from the woman in whom the fertilization took place to another woman.

Infertility: the inability of a couple to achieve a pregnancy after one year of regular unprotected sexual relations or the inability of the woman to carry a pregnancy to a live birth.

IUD: abbreviation for intrauterine device, a birth control measure.

Karyotype: appearance of chromosomes, including their size, number, and shape.

Klinefelter's syndrome: a congenital abnormality of the male wherein his sex chromosome type is XXY instead of XY.

Laparoscopy: direct visualization of the ovaries and the exterior of the fallopian tubes and uterus by means of an instrument introduced through a small incision below the navel; can be accompanied by egg removal via an instrument introduced through another small incision to puncture the ovarian follicle and suck out an egg.

Laparotomy: surgical procedure to explore the abdominal cavity or repair reproductive organs.

Luteal phase: second part of a woman's menstrual cycle, after the release of an egg from the ovary.

Lutenizing hormone (LH): a hormone secreted by the pituitary throughout the menstrual cycle, with a "peak" just prior to ovulation.

Microsurgery: surgery that is performed while the physician is observing the bodily structure being operated on through a microscope.

Miscarriage: a spontaneous abortion of a fetus prior to viability.

Morphology of sperm: shape and structure of sperm.

Motility of sperm: the ability of sperm to move.

Mumps orchitis: inflammation of the testicle caused by the mumps virus.

Obstetrician: a physician who supervises pregnancy and childbirth.

Oligospermia: scarcity of sperm in the semen.

Oocyte: see *ovum.*

Ova: plural of ovum.

Ovaries: the two female sexual glands in which the eggs are developed and the hormones estrogen and progesterone are produced.

Oviduct: fallopian tube.

Ovulation: the discharge of an egg, generally around the midpoint of the menstrual cycle.

Ovum: the reproductive cell (egg) produced monthly in the ovaries.

Pelvic inflammatory disease (PID): inflammatory disease of the pelvis, often caused by an infection.

Penis: the male organ of intercourse.

Peritoneal cavity: abdominal cavity.

Peritoneum: membrane lining the abdominal cavity.

Peritonitis: inflammation of the membrane lining the abdominal cavity.

Pituitary: a gland at the base of the brain that secretes a number of hormones related to fertility.

Polycystic ovaries: development of multiple cysts in the ovaries, presumably due to a failure of the ovaries to expel eggs.

Polygenic: caused by a combination of genes.

Postcoital test: the analysis, under a microscope, of vaginal and cervical secretions within several hours of sexual relations.

Premature ejaculation: discharge of sperm from the penis prior to or immediately after entering the vagina.

Progesterone: a hormone secreted by the ovary after ovulation has occurred.

Prostate gland: male gland that supplies part of the fluid of the semen.

Reanastomose: to rejoin.

Recessive genetic defect: abnormality which manifests itself when both genes in a gene pair are defective.

Retrograde ejaculation: discharge of sperm backward into the bladder rather than out through the penis.

Retroverted uterus: uterus that is flexed severely forward or backward.

Rubin test: the administration of carbon dioxide gas into the uterus and fallopian tube to determine if the tubes are open.

Salpingitis: inflammation of the fallopian tubes.

Salpingolysis: surgery to clear the fallopian tubes of adhesions.

Salpingoplasty: surgery to correct blocked fallopian tubes.

Scrotum: sac that contains the male testicles.

Secondary infertility: the inability to conceive or carry a pregnancy after having successfully conceived and carried one or more pregnancies.

Semen: the secretions ejaculated during orgasm, which include sperm.

Semen analysis: the microscopic evaluation of the ejaculate to determine the number of sperm per cubic centimeter, their shape, their size, and their ability to move.

Seminiferous tubules: small tubes in the testicles where sperm are formed.

Sims-Huhner test: see *postcoital test*.

Sperm bank: place in which sperm is stored frozen for future use in artificial insemination by donor or by husband.

Spermatogenesis: the creation of sperm.

Stein-Leventhal disease: polycystic ovaries.

Stillbirth: the birth of a dead fetus.

Surrogate carrier: woman who gestates an embryo which is not genetically related to her and then turns over the child to its genetic parents.

Surrogate mother: a woman who becomes pregnant through insemination with the sperm of the husband of an infertile woman and then turns the child over for adoption by the couple.

Test tube baby: child born through *in vitro* fertilization.

Testes: plural of testicle.

Testicle: the two male sexual glands in which sperm and the male hormone testosterone are produced.

Testicular biopsy: small surgical excision of testicular tissue to determine whether sperm are being produced.

Testosterone: a male sex hormone, produced in the testicles.

Tubal ligation: sterilization of a woman by excision of a small segment of each fallopian tube.

Tubal cautery: sterilization of a woman by sealing the fallopian tubes with heat.

Tuboplasty: surgical repair of the fallopian tubes.

Turner's syndrome: a congenital abnormality of the female wherein her sex chromosomal type is XO instead of XX.

Ultrasound: a sonar device which can be used to bounce sound waves off the abdomen of a woman with the waves being translated into a TV screen picture of her inner abdomen to view such things as an ovarian follicle or a fetus.

Urethra: the passage that carries urine from the bladder; in the male, it also carries semen from the prostate to the point of ejaculation.

Urologist: a physician who specializes in diseases of the urinary tract in men and women and of the reproductive organs in men.

Uterus: the organ which houses and nourishes the fetus from implantation until birth.

Vagina: the female organ of intercourse and the opening through which a baby travels out of the uterus in the process of being born.

Varicocele: a varicose vein of the spermatic cord in the testicle.

Vas deferens: the convoluted duct that carries sperm from the testicle to the ejaculatory duct of the penis.

Vasectomy: surgery to excise part of the vas deferens to sterilize a man.

Vasogram: X ray of sperm ducts.

Venereal disease: any infection transmitted by sexual intercourse.

Wedge resection: surgical procedure in which a small section is cut out of the ovary and the ovary is then sutured together.

Wrongful birth lawsuit: legal case brought by parents of a genetically defective child claiming that a physician or laboratory failed to explain genetic risks or incorrectly performed genetic tests.

Wrongful life lawsuit: legal case brought in the name of a genetically defective child claiming that a physician or laboratory failed to explain genetic risks or incorrectly performed genetic tests.

❦ APPENDIX C

Resources

March of Dimes Birth Defects Foundation
1275 Mamaroneck Avenue
White Plains, NY 10605

Provides information on genetic counseling and testing and referrals to physicians and genetics centers; has local chapters across the country.

National Genetics Foundation
555 West 57th Street
New York, NY 10019

Provides information on genetic counseling and testing and referrals.

RESOLVE, Inc.
Post Office Box 474
Belmont, MA 02178-0474

A national self-help group for infertile couples that has 43 volunteer-run chapters around the country providing referrals, support groups, and literature. The national headquarters provides many services including telephone counseling, medical consultation, a periodic newsletter, and information about all aspects of infertility and its treatment.

American Fertility Society
1608 13th Avenue South, Suite 101
Birmingham, AL 35256-6199

The national organization of infertility specialists, providing referrals to physicians and publishing some literature for a lay audience (as well as *Fertility and Sterility,* a medical journal).

The Barren Foundation
60 East Monroe Street
Chicago, IL 60603

Presents medical seminars, holds support groups, and provides a directory of infertility specialists and literature on infertility.

American College of Obstetricians and Gynecologists
600 Maryland Avenue S.W., Suite 300
Washington, DC 20024

Provides referrals to board-certified infertility specialists.

American Association of Tissue Banks
12111 Parklawn Drive
Rockville, MD 20852

This organization's Reproductive Council has developed standards for sperm banks.

Donors Offspring
Post Office Box 33
Sarcoxie, MO 64862

For AID children searching for their donor/fathers.

International Soundex Reunion Registry
Post Office Box 2312
Carson City, NV 89701

For AID children searching for their donor/fathers.

Center for Communications in Infertility, Inc.
Post Office Box 516
Yorktown Heights, NY 10598

Publishes a bimonthly newsletter, *PERSPECTIVES on Infertility,* and provides information on infertility specialists, counselors, artificial insemination, support groups, *in vitro* fertilization clinics, and surrogate motherhood.

Surrogate Parenting News
120 North Fourth Avenue
Ann Arbor, MI 48104

A monthly publication about legal and medical issues in surrogate motherhood, artificial insemination, and *in vitro* fertilization.

❧ APPENDIX D
Selected Readings on Medical, Legal, and Ethical Aspects of the New Conceptions

IN VITRO FERTILIZATION, EMBRYO TRANSFER, AND EMBRYO FREEZING

- **SELECTED MEDICAL PUBLICATIONS:**

Don P. Wolf and Martin M. Quigley, *Human In Vitro Fertilization and Embryo Transfer* (Plenum Press, forthcoming).

J.E. Buster *et al.*, "Non-surgical Transfer of *In Vivo* Fertilized Donated Ova to Five Infertile Women: Report of Two Pregnancies," 2 *Lancet* 223 (1983).

"Selected Reprints: Infertility Therapy with a Special Focus on In Vitro Fertilization," *Fertility and Sterility* (April 1983).

Alan Trounson, John Leeton, Mandy Besanko, Carl Wood and Angelo Conti, "Pregnancy Established in An Infertile Patient After Transfer of a Donated Embryo Fertilised In Vitro," 286 *British Medical Journal* 835 (1983).

Howard W. Jones *et al.* "The Program for *In Vitro Fertilization* at Norfolk," 38 *Fertility and Sterility* 14 (1982).

John D. Biggers, "In Vitro Fertilization and Embryo Transfer in Human Beings," 304 *New England Journal of Medicine* 336 (1981).

Luigi Mastroianni, *et al.* eds., *Fertilization and Embryonic Development In Vitro* (1981).

R. G. Edwards, P. C. Steptoe, and J. M. Purdy, "Establishing Full-term Human Pregnancies Using Cleaving Embryos Grown *In Vitro*," 87 *British Journal of Obstetrics and Gynaecology* 737 (1980).

Alexander Lopata, Ian W. H. Johnston, Ian J. Hoult, and Andrew I. Speirs, "Pregnancy Following Intrauterine Implantation of an Embryo Obtained by *In Vitro* Fertilization of a Preovulatory Egg," 33 *Fertility and Sterility* 117 (1980).

Pierre Soupart, "Current Status of In Vitro Fertilization and Embryo Transfer in Man," 23 *Clinical Obstetrics and Gynecology* 683 (1980).

Laurence E. Karp and Roger P. Donahue, "Preimplantation Ectogenesis: Science and Speculation Concerning *In Vitro* Fertilization and Related Procedures," 124 *Western Journal of Medicine* 282 (1976).

• **CASES**

Del Zio v. Manhattan's Columbia Presbyterian Medical Center, No. 74-3558. (S.D.N.Y. filed April 12, 1978);

Smith v. Fahner, No. 82 c 4324 (N.D.Ill., memorandum opinion February 4, 1983).

In Vitro Fertilization Statutes:

Ill. Rev. Stat. ch. 38 §81-26(7) (1981).

Pa. Stat. Ann. tit. 18 §3213(e) (Supp. 1983-84).

• **FETAL RESEARCH STATUTES POSSIBLY AFFECTING IN VITRO FERTILIZATION, EMBRYO TRANSFER, OR EMBRYO FREEZING (* Indicates that statute explicitly extends to research on embryos; † Indicates that the statute only covers research in conjunction with an abortion):**

*†   Ariz. Rev. Stat. Ann §36-2302 (Supp. 1982-83);

*†   Cal. Health & Safety Code §25956 (West Supp. 1983);

*†   Ill. Ann. Stat. ch. 38 §81-26, §81-32, -32.1 (Smith-Hurd Supp. 1983-84);

†   Ind. Code §35-1-58.5-6 (1979);

*†   Ky. Rev. Stat. Ann. §436.026 (1975);

*   La. Rev. Stat. Ann. §14:87.2 (West 1974);

    Me. Rev. Stat. Ann. tit. 22 §1593 (West 1980);

*   Mass. Ann. Laws ch. 112 §12J (Michie/Law Co-op Supp. 1982);

*   Mich. Comp. Laws Ann. §§333.2685 - .2692 (West 1980);

*   Minn. Stat. Ann. §145.421 - .422 (West Supp. 1982);

*   Mo. Ann. Stat. §188.037 (Vernon Supp. 1983);

    Mont. Code Ann. §50-20-108(3) (1981);

†   Neb. Rev. Stat. §28-342, 28-346 (1979);

*   N. M. Stat. Ann. §24-9A-1 et seq (1981);

*   N. D. Cent. Code §14-02.2-01 to -02 (Allen Smith 1981);

*†   Ohio Rev. Code Ann. §2919.14 (Baldwin 1982);

*†   Okla. Stat. Ann. tit. 63 §1-735 (West Supp. 1982-83);

*†   Pa. Stat. Ann. tit. 18 §3216 (Purdon Supp. 1983-84);

*   R. I. Gen. Laws §11-54-2 (Supp. 1982);

       S. D. Comp. Laws Ann. §34-23A-17 (1977);

†   Tenn. Code Ann. §39-4-208 (1982);

       Utah Code Ann. §76-7-310 (Allen Smith 1978);

†   Wyo. Stat. 35-6-115 (1977);

• *SELECTED LEGAL PUBLICATIONS:*

George J. Annas and Sherman Elias, "*In Vitro* Fertilization and Embryo Transfer: Medicolegal Aspects of a New Technique to Create a Family," 17 *Family Law Quarterly* 199 (1983).

Kathryn Venturatos Lorio, "In Vitro Fertilization and Embryo Transfer: Fertile Areas for Litigation," 35 *Southwestern Law Journal* 973 (1982).

Comment, "New Reproductive Technologies: The Legal Problem and a Solution," 49 *Tennessee Law Review* 303 (1982).

Comment, "Love's Labor Lost: Legal and Ethical Implications in Artificial Human Procreation," 58 *Journal of Urban Law* 459 (1981).

Bernard M. Dickens, "The Ectogenic Human Being: A Problem Child of our Time," 18 *University of Western Ontario Law Review* 241 (1980).

Barbara F. Katz, "Legal Implications & Regulation of *In Vitro* Fertilization," *Genetics and the Law II* 351 (ed. by Aubrey Milunsky and George J. Annas) (1980).

Dennis M. Flannery, Carol Drescher Weisman, Christopher R. Lipsett, Alan N. Braverman, "Test Tube Babies: Legal Issues Raised by *In Vitro* Fertilization," 67 *Georgetown Law Journal* 1295 (1979).

Comment, "Lawmaking & Science: A Practical Look at In Vitro Fertilization and Embryo Transfer," III *Detroit College of Law Review* 429 (1979).

Douglas J. Cuisine, "Some Legal Implications of Embryo Transfer," 129 *New Law Journal* 627 (1979).

Comment, "Artificial Human Reproduction: Legal Problems Presented by the Test Tube Baby," 28 *Emory Law Journal* 1045 (1979).

Mark E. Cohen, "The 'Brave New Baby' & the Law: Fashioning Remedies for the Victims of *In Vitro* Fertilization," 4 *American Journal of Law & Medicine* 319 (1978).

Dennis J. Tuchler, "Man Made Man and the Law," 22 *St. Louis University Law Journal* 310 (1978).

Philip Reilly, "In Vitro Fertilization—A Legal Perspective," *Genetics and the Law* 359 (ed. by Aubrey Milunsky and George J. Annas) (1976).

Kevin Abel, "The Legal Implications of Ectogenic Research," 10 *University of Tulsa Law Journal* 243 (1974).

• *OTHER RESOURCES:*

Peter Singer and William A. W. Walters, eds., *Test Tube Babies* (1982).

Clifford Grobstein, *From Chance to Purpose: An Appraisal of External Human Fertilization* (1981).

Robert Edwards and Patrick Steptoe, *A Matter of Life* (1980).

Ethics Advisory Board, *Report and Conclusions: HEW Support of Research Involving Human In Vitro Fertilization and Embryo Transfer* (1979).

Lesley and John Brown, *Our Miracle Called Louise* (1979).

ARTIFICIAL INSEMINATION

• *SELECTED MEDICAL PUBLICATIONS:*

William Beck and E. Wallach, "When Therapy Fails—Artificial Insemination," 17 *Contemporary OB/GYN* 114 (No. 1, 1981).

Martin Curie-Cohen, Lesleigh Luttrell, and Sander Shapiro, "Current Practice of Artificial Insemination by Donor in the United States," 300 *New England Journal of Medicine* 585 (1979).

Melvin L. Taymor, "Therapeutic Donor Insemination," *Infertility* 204 (1978).

Richard D. Amelar and Lawrence Dubin, "Artificial Donor Insemination (AID)" in Richard D. Amelar, Lawrence Dubin, Patrick C. Walsh, *Male Infertility* 237 (1977).

Barbara and Allen Harvey, "How Couples Feel About Donor Insemination," 9 *Contemporary OB/GYN* 93 (No. 6, 1977).

"Techniques of Artificial Insemination," 9 *Contemporary OB/GYN* 63 (No. 6, 1977).

Wilfred Finegold, *Artificial Insemination* (1976).

William W. Beck, Jr., "A Critical Look at the Legal, Ethical and Technical Aspects of Artificial Insemination," 27 *Fertility and Sterility* 1 (1976).

Amnon David and Dalia Avidan, "Artificial Insemination Donor: Clinical and Psychologic Aspects," 27 *Fertility and Sterility* 528 (1976).

David P. Goldstein, "Artificial Insemination by Donor—Status and Problems," *Genetics and the Law* 197 (ed. by Aubrey Milunsky and George J. Annas) (1976).

Richard E. Dixon and Veasy Buttram, "Artificial Insemination Using Donor Semen: A Review of 171 Cases," 27 *Fertility and Sterility* 130 (1976).

J. K. Sherman, "Synopsis of the Use of Frozen Human Semen Since 1964: State of the Art of Human Semen Banking," 24 *Fertility and Sterility* 397 (1973).

Keith D. Smith and Emil Steinberger, "Survival of Spermatozoa in a Human Bank," 223 *Journal of the American Medical Association* 774 (1973).

• *CASES:*

Fitzgerald v. Rueckl, No. 300171 (Washoe County, Nevada, 2d Judicial Court, filed October 20, 23, 1978, appeal dismissed January 28, 1982).

R. S. v. G. S. (Superior Court of New Jersey, Hunterdon County, January 6, 1982), *Reporter on Human Reproduction and the Law,* January-February, 1982.

C.M. v. C.C., 377 A. 2d 821, 152 N.J. Super. 160 (1977);

In re Adoption of Anonymous, 74 Misc. 2d 99, 345 N.Y.S. 2d 430 (Kings County, New York, Surrogate's Court, 1973);

People v. Sorenson, 68 Cal 2d 280, 437 P 2d 495, 66 Cal Rptr 7 (1968);

Anonymous v. Anonymous, 41 Misc. 2d 886, 246 N.Y.S. 2d 406 (Kings County, New York, Supreme Court, 1964);

Gursky v. Gursky, 39 Misc. 2d 1083, 242 N.Y.S. 2d 406 (Kings County, New York, Supreme Court, 1963);

People ex. rel. Abajian v. Dennett, 15 Misc. 2d 260, 184 N.Y.S. 2d 178 (New York County, New York, Supreme Court, 1956);

Doornbos v. Doornbos, 23 U.S.L.W. 2308 (Cook County, Illinois, Superior Court, December 13, 1954), appeal dismissed on procedural grounds, 12 Ill. App. 2d 473, 139 N.E. 2d 844 (1956);

Strnad v. Strnad, 190 Misc. 786, 78 N.Y.S. 2d 390 (New York County, New York, Supreme Court, 1948).

• *STATUTES:*

Alaska Stat. §25.20.045 (Supp. 1982);

Ark. Stat. Ann. §61-141 (1971);

Cal. Civ. Code §7005 (West Supp. 1983);

Colo. Rev. Stat. §19-6-106 (1978);

Conn. Gen. Stat. §§45-69f to -69n (1981);

Fla. Stat. Ann. §742.11 (West Supp. 1983);

Ga. Code Ann. §§74-101.1, -9904 (1982);

Kan. Stat. Ann. §§23-128 to -130 (1981);

La. Civ. Code Ann. art. 188 (West Supp. 1983);

Md. Est. & Trusts Code Ann. §1-206(b) (1974); and Md. Health-General Ann. Code §20-214 (1982);

Mich. Comp. Laws Ann. §333.2824 (1980) and §700.111 (1980);

Minn. Stat. Ann. §257.56;

Mont. Rev. Code Ann. §40-6-106 (1981);

Nev. Rev. Stat. §126.061 (1979);

N. Y. Dom. Rel. Law §73 (McKinney 1977);

N. C. Gen. Stat. §49A-1 (1976);

Okla. Stat. Ann. tit. 10, §§551-553 (West Supp. 1982-1983);

Or. Rev. Stat. §§109.239, .243, .247, 677.355, .360, .365, 370 (1981);

Tenn. Code Ann. § 53-446 (Supp. 1981);

Tex. Fam. Code Ann. §12.03 (Vernon 1975);

Va. Code §64.1-7.1 (1980);

Wash. Rev. Code Ann. §26.26.050 (West Supp. 1983-1984);

Wis. Stat. Ann §767.47(9) (West 1981), §891.40 (West Supp. 1982-1983).

Wyo. Stat. §14-2-103 (1978).

• *SELECTED LEGAL PUBLICATIONS:*

George P. Smith, "Artificial Insemination Redivivus: Permutations Within a Penumbra," 2 *Journal of Legal Medicine* 113 (1981).

Barbara Kritchevsky, "The Unmarried Woman's Right to Artificial Insemination: A Call for an Expanded Definition of Family," 4 *Harvard Woman's Law Journal* 1 (1981).

Note, "Eugenic Artificial Insemination: A Cure for Mediocrity?" 94 *Harvard Law Review* 1850 (1981).

Jeffrey M. Shaman, "Legal Aspects of Artificial Insemination," 18 *Journal of Family Law* 331 (1979-80).

Note, "Artificial Insemination: A Legislative Remedy," 3 *Western State University Law Review* 48 (1975).

Comment, "Artificial Insemination: Problems, Policies and Proposals," 26 *Alabama Law Review* 120 (1973).

Charles P. Kindregan, "State Power Over Human Fertility and Individual Liberty," 23 *Hastings Law Journal* 1401 (1972).

Winthrop P. Thies, "A Look to the Future: Property Rights and the Posthumously Conceived Child," 110 *Trust & Estates* 922 (1971).

Note, "Therapeutic Impregnation: Prognosis of a Lawyer—Diagnosis of a Legislature," 39 *University of Cincinnati Law Review* 291 (1970).

Walter Wadlington, "Artificial Insemination: The Dangers of a Poorly Kept Secret," 64 *Northwestern University Law Review* 777 (1970).

• *OTHER RESOURCES:*

American Fertility Society, *Report of the Ad Hoc Committee on Artificial Insemination* (1980).

"Reproductive Council Guidelines," 4 *American Association of Tissue Banks Newsletter* 37 (November 1980).

S. J. Behrman, "Artificial Insemination and Public Policy," 300 *New England Journal of Medicine* 619 (1979).

Mark S. Frankel, "Artificial Insemination and Semen Cryobanking: Health and Safety Concerns and the Role of Professional Standards, Law and Public Policy," 3 *Legal Medical Quarterly* 93 (1979).

SURROGATE MOTHERHOOD

• *CASES:*

In Re: Baby Girl, No. 83AD (Jefferson County, Kentucky, Circuit Court, Sixth Division, March 8, 1983), 9 *Family Law Reporter* 2348 (April 5, 1983).

Syrkowski v. Appleyard, Civ. Action 81 122 683 DP (Wayne County, Michigan Circuit Court, November 25, 1981), affirmed, 9 *Family Law Reporter* 2260–61 (March 1, 1983).

Commonwealth vs. Surrogate Parenting Assocs., Inc., No. 81-CI-0429, (Franklin County, Kentucky, Circuit Court Division 1, filed March 12, 1981), 7 *Family Law Reporter* 2246 (Feb. 17, 1981).

Doe v. Kelley, 6 *Family Law Reporter* 3011 (Wayne County, Michigan, Circuit Court, January 28, 1980), affirmed 106 Mich. App. 169, 307 N.W. 2d 438 (1981).

Noyes v. Thrane, No. CF 7614 (Los Angeles County, California, Superior Court, filed Feb. 20, 1981).

Attorney General Opinions:

"Surrogate Motherhood Contracts Declared Illegal by Kentucky A. G.," 7 *Family Law Reporter* 2246, 2247 (1981).

• *STATUTES THAT PROHIBIT PAYMENT IN CONNECTION WITH AN ADOPTION (* Indicates that the statute exempts stepparents from the expense reporting requirements):*

*   Ala. Code §26-10-8 (1975);

*   Ariz. Rev. Stat. Ann. §8-126 (c) (1974);

*   California Penal Code §273 (a) (West 1970);

Colo. Rev. Stat. §19-4-115 (1978);

Del. Code Ann. tit. 13 §928 (1981);

*   Fla. Stat. Ann. §63.212 (1) (b) (West Supp. 1983);

Ga. Code Ann. §74-418 (b) (Supp 1982);

Idaho Code §18-1511 (1979);

*   Ill. Ann. Stat. ch. 40 §§1526, 1701, 1702 (Smith Hurd 1980);

Iowa Code Ann. §600.9 (West 1981);

Ky. Rev. Stat. §199.590 (2) (1982);

Md. Ann. Code art. 16 §83 (1981);

Mass. Ann. Laws ch. 210 §11A (1981);

Mich. Comp. Laws Ann. §710.54 (West Supp. 1983-84);

Nev. Rev. Stat. §127.290 (1981);

*   N.J. Stat. Ann. §9:3-54 (West Supp. 1983-84);

N.Y. Soc. Serv. Law §374 (6) (McKinney Supp. 1982-83);

N.C. Gen. Stat. §48-37 (Supp. 1981);

S.D. Codified Laws Ann. §25-6-4.2 (Supp. 1982);

Tenn. Code Ann. §36-136 (Supp. 1982);

Utah Code Ann. §76-7-203 (1978);

Wis. Stat. Ann. §946.716 (1982).

• *SELECTED LEGAL PUBLICATIONS:*

Ralph D. Mawdsley, "Surrogate Parenthood: A Need for Legislative Direction," 7 *Illinois Bar Journal* 412 (1983).

William W. Handel and Bernard A. Sherwyn, "Surrogate Parenting," 18 *Trial* 57 (1982).

Lisa J. Greenberg and Harold L. Hirsch, "Surrogate Motherhood and Artificial Insemination: Contractual Implications," 29 *Medical Trial Technique Quarterly* 149 (1982).

M. Louise Graham, "Surrogate Gestation and the Protection of Choice," 22 *Santa Clara Law Review* 291 (1982).

Note, "The Surrogate Mother Contract in Indiana," 15 *Indiana Law Review* 807 (1982).

C. A. Rushevsky, "Legal Recognition of Surrogate Gestation," 7 *Women's Rights Law Reporter* 107 (1982).

Comment, "Surrogate Motherhood: The Attorney's Legal and Ethical Dilemma," 11 *Capitol University Law Review* 593 (1982).

Comment, "Surrogate Mother Agreements: Contemporary Legal Aspects of A Biblical Notion," 16 *University of Richmond Law Review* 467, (1982).

James Edward Maule, "Federal Tax Consequences of Surrogate Motherhood," *Taxes* 656 (September 1982).

Comment, "Parenthood by Proxy: Legal Implications of Surrogate Birth," 67 *Iowa Law Review* 385 (1982).

Katie Marie Brophy, "A Surrogate Mother Contract to Bear a Child," 20 *Journal of Family Law* 263 (1981-82).

Comment, "Artificial Insemination and Surrogate Motherhood—A Nursery Full of Unresolved Questions," 17 *Willamette Law Review* 913 (1981).

Note, "Surrogate Motherhood: The Outer Limits of Protected Conduct," IV *Detroit College of Law Review* 1131 (1981).

Note, "Surrogate Mothers: The Legal Issues," 7 *American Journal of Law and Medicine* 323 (1981).

Note, "Surrogate Mothering: Medical Reality in a Legal Vacuum," 8 *Journal of Legislation* 140 (1981).

Lori B. Andrews, "Removing the Stigma of Surrogate Motherhood," 4 *Family Advocate* 20 (No. 2, 1981).

Comment, "Surrogate Motherhood in California: Legislative Proposals," 18 *San Diego Law Review* 341 (1981).

Note, "In Defense of Surrogate Parenting: A Critical Analysis of the Recent Kentucky Experience," 69 *Kentucky Law Journal* 877 (1980-81).

Noel P. Keane, "Legal Problems of Surrogate Motherhood," 1980 *Southern Illinois University Law Journal* 147.

Comment, "Contracts to Bear a Child," 66 *California Law Review* 611 (1978).

• **OTHER RESOURCES:**

Noel P. Keane with Dennis L. Breo, *The Surrogate Mother* (1981).

GENETIC COUNSELING, TESTING AND ENGINEERING

• **SELECTED PUBLICATIONS WITH MEDICAL AND COUNSELING INFORMATION:**

American Society of Law and Medicine, *Biological Monitoring and Genetic Screening in the Workplace* (conference materials) (May 1983).

President's Commission for the Study of Ethical Problems in Medicine and Biomedical and Behavioral Research, *Screening and Counseling for Genetic Conditions: The Ethical, Social and Legal Implications of Genetic Screening, Counseling, and Education Programs* (1983).

James Le Fanu, "Fetal Diagnosis of Thalasemia," 24 *Medical Tribune* 1 (March 2, 1983).

Committee on Genetics, "New Issues in Newborn Screening for Phenylketonuria and Congenital Hypothryoidism," 69 *Pediatrics* 1 (1982).

Joe L. Simpson, *Genetics in Obstetrics and Gynecology* (1982).

John C. Fletcher, *Coping With Genetic Disorders: A Guide for Counseling* (1982).

P. Ryder and A. Svejgaard, "Genetics of HLA Disease Association," 15 *Annual Review of Genetics* 169 (1981).

H. Eldon Sutton, *An Introduction to Human Genetics, 3rd Edition* (1980).

James S. Thompson and Margaret W. Thompson, *Genetics in Medicine, 3rd Edition* (1980).

B. Cohen, *et al.*, eds., *Genetic Issues in Public Health and Medicine* (1979).

A. M. Capron, *et al.*, eds., *Genetic Counseling: Facts, Values and Norms* (1979).

G. Evers-Kiebooms and H. van den Bergil, "Impact of Genetic Counseling: A Review of Published Follow-Up Studies," 15 *Clinical Genetics* 465 (1979).

National Institute of Child Health and Human Development, *Antenatal Diagnosis: Report of a Consensus Development Conference* (1979).

Aubrey Milunsky, *Know Your Genes* (1978).

H. Lubs, ed., *Genetic Counseling* (1977).

Laurence E. Karp, *Genetic Engineering: Threat or Promise?* (1976).

Committee for the Study of Inborn Errors of Metabolism, National Academy of Sciences, *Genetic Screening: Programs, Principles and Research* (1975).

Victor A. McKusick, *Mendelian Inheritance in Man: Catalogs of Autosomal Dominant, Autosomal Recessive, & X-Linked Phenotypes* (5th edition, 1975).

Mack Lipkin, Jr., and Peter T. Rowley, eds., *Genetic Responsibility: On Choosing Our Children's Genes* (1974).

Claire O. Leonard, Gary A. Chase and Barton Childs, "Genetic Counseling: A Consumer's View," 287 *New England Journal of Medicine* 433 (1972).

A. Stevenson, V. Davison, and M. Oakes, *Genetic Counseling* (1970).

• *CASES:*

Harbeson v. Parke-Davis, Inc. 98 Wash. 2d 460, 656 P. 2d 483 (1983).

Turpin v. Sortini, 31 Cal. 3d 220, 233, 182 Cal. Rptr. 337, 345, 643 P. 2d 954 (1982).

Naccash v. Burger, 290 S.E. 2d 825 (Va 1982).

Schroeder v. Perkel, 87 N.J. 53, 432 A. 2d 834 (1981).

Robak v. United States, 658 F. 2d 471 (7th Cir. 1981).

Eisbrenner v. Stanley, 106 Mich. App. 357, 308 N.W. 2d 209 (1981).

Speck v. Finegold, 439 A. 2d 110 (1981).

Phillips v. United States, 508 F. Supp. 537 (D.S.C. 1980).

Curlender v. Bio-Science Laboratories 106 Cal. App. 3d 811, 165 Cal. Rptr. 477 (Cal. Ct. App. 1980).

Berman v. Allen, 80 N.J. 421, 404 A. 2d 8 (1979).

Becker v. Schwartz, 46 N.Y. 2d 401, 386 N.E. 2d 807 (1978).

Dumer v. St. Michael's Hospital, 69 Wis. 2d 766, 233 N.W. 3d 372 (1975).

Jacobs v. Theimer, 519 S.W. 2d 846 (1975).

• *SELECTED LEGAL PUBLICATIONS:*

Comment, "Wrongful Birth and Wrongful Life: Questions of Public Policy," 28 *Loyola Law Review* 77 (1982).

Note, "Child v. Parent: A Viable New Tort of Wrongful Life?" 24 *Arizona Law Review* 391 (1982).

Note, "Preference for Nonexistence: Wrongful Life and a Proposed Tort for Genetic Malpractice," 55 *Southern California Law Review* 477 (1982).

"Selected Materials on Wrongful Life—Birth," 37 *The Record of the Association of the Bar of the City of New York* 583 (1982).

Thomas DeWitt Rogers III, "Wrongful Life and Wrongful Birth: Medical Malpractice in Genetic Counseling and Prenatal Testing," 33 *South Carolina Law Review* 713 (1982).

Comment, "Damages in Genetic Mutation and Chromosomal Breakage: Tort Actions," 25 *St. Louis University Law Journal* 105 (1981).

Comment, "Liability for Negligent Prenatal Diagnosis: Parents' Right to a 'Perfect Child'?" 42 *Ohio State Law Journal* 551 (1981).

Note, "Wrongful Birth: A Child of Tort Comes of Age," 50 *University of Cincinnati Law Review* 65 (1981).

Note, "Reassessment of 'Wrongful Life' and 'Wrongful Birth,'" 1980 *Wisconsin Law Review* 782 (1980).

Alexander Morgan Capron, "Tort Liability and Genetic Counseling," 79 *Columbia Law Review* 618 (1979).

Constance Gould and Ted Stiles, "The Prevention of Mental Retardation: The Physician's Changing Standard of Care and the Need for Legislative Action," 13 *Gonzaga Law Review* 691 (1978).

Note, "Father and Mother Know Best: Defining the Liability of Physicians for Inadequate Genetic Counseling," 87 *Yale Law Journal* 1488 (1978).

Note, "Wrongful Birth Damages: Mandate and Mishandling by Judicial Fiat," 13 *Valparaiso University Law Review* 127 (1978).

Joseph S. Kashi, "The Case of the Unwanted Blessing: Wrongful Life," 31 *University of Miami Law Journal* 1409 (1977).

Note, "Wrongful Birth and Emotional Distress Damages: A Suggested Approach," 38 *University of Pittsburgh Law Review* 550 (1977).

George J. Annas and Brian Coyne, "Fitness for Birth and Reproduction: Legal Implications of Genetic Screening," 9 *Family Law Quarterly* 463 (1975).

Note, "Fetal Research: A View from Right to Life to Wrongful Birth," 52 *Chicago Kent Law Review* 133 (1975).

• *OTHER RESOURCES:*

Zsolt Harsanyi and Richard Hutton, *Genetic Prophecy: Beyond the Double Helix* (1981).

U.S. Department of Health and Human Services, *State Laws and Regulations on Genetic Disorders* (July 1980), DHHS Pub. No. (HSA) 81-5243.

Aubrey Milunsky and George J. Annas, eds., *Genetics and the Law* II (1980).

Marc Lappé, *Genetic Politics* (1979).

Tabitha M. Powledge and John Fletcher, "Guidelines for the Ethical, Social and Legal Issues in Prenatal Diagnosis," 300 *New England Journal of Medicine* 168 (1979).

Philip Reilly, *Genetics, Law and Social Policy* (1977).

M. Lappé *et al.*, "Ethical and Social Issues in Screening for Genetic Disease," 286 *New England Journal of Medicine* 1129 (1972).

ETHICS OF THE NEW CONCEPTIONS

Beverly Freeman, "Facing the Ethical Issues," *Resolve Newsletter* 1 (June 1983).

Hans. O. Tiefel, "Human In Vitro Fertilization," 247 *Journal of the American Medical Association* 3235 (1982).

Alan O. Trounson, Carl Wood and John F. Leeton, "Freezing of Embryos: An Ethical Obligation," 2 *Medical Journal of Australia* 332 (1982).

J. Kerby Anderson, *Genetic Engineering* (1982).

LeRoy Walters, "Human In Vitro Fertilization: A Review of the Ethical Literature," 9 (4) *Hastings Center Report* 23 (August 1979).

Leon Kass, "'Making Babies' Revisited," 54 *Public Interest* 32 (1979).

Joseph Fletcher, *The Ethics of Genetics Control: Ending Reproductive Roulette* (1974).

R. G. Edwards, "Fertilization of Human Eggs In Vitro: Morals, Ethics & the Law," 49 *Quarterly Review of Biology* 3 (1974).

Paul Ramsey, "Shall We 'Reproduce'? I. The Medical Ethics of In Vitro Fertilization," 220 *Journal of the American Medical Association* 1346 (1972).

Paul Ramsey, "Shall We 'Reproduce'? II. Rejoinders and Future Forecast," 220 *Journal of the American Medical Association* 1480 (1972).

Leon Kass, "Making Babies—the New Biology and the 'Old' Morality," 26 *Public Interest* 32 (1972).

Robert G. Edward and David J. Sharpe, "Social Values and Research in Human Embryology," 231 *Nature* 87 (1971).

James D. Watson, "Moving Toward Clonal Man—Is This What We Want?" 117 *Congressional Record* 12751 (1971).

Paul Ramsey, *Fabricated Man: The Ethics of Genetic Control* (1970).

GENERAL RESOURCES ON NEW CONCEPTIONS

Walter Wadlington, "Artificial Conception: The Challenge for Family Law," 69 *Virginia Law Review* 465 (1983).

Lori B. Andrews, "Embryo Technology," *Parents* 63 (May 1981).

Ciba Foundation Symposium, *Law and Ethics of A.I.D. and Embryo Transfer* (1973).

Robert T. Francoeur, *Utopian Motherhood: New Trends in Human Reproduction* (1970).

GENERAL INFERTILITY RESOURCES

Patricia Harper and Jan Aitken, *A Child is Not the "Cure" for Infertility* (1982).

Edward E. Wallach and Roger D. Kempers, *Modern Trends in Infertility and Conception Control* (1982).

Rochelle Friedman and Bonnie Gradstein, *Surviving Pregnancy Loss* (1982).

Sherman J. Silber, *How to Get Pregnant* (1981).

Susan Borg and Judith Lasker, *When Pregnancy Fails: Families Coping with Miscarriage, Stillbirth, and Infant Death* (1981).

Mary Harrison, *Infertility: A Guide for Couples* (1979).

John J. Stangel, *Fertility and Conception: An Essential Guide for Childless Couples* (1979).

Melvin Taymor, *Infertility* (1978).

International Planned Parenthood Federation, ed., *Handbook on Infertility* (1977).

Barbara Eck Menning, *Infertility: A Guide for the Childless Couple* (1977).

Richard D. Amelar, Lawrence Dubin and Patrick C. Walsh, eds., *Male Infertility* (1977).

A. T. K. Cockett and Ronald L. Urry, eds., *Male Infertility: Workup, Treatment and Research* (1977).

S. J. Behrman and Robert W. Kistner, *Progress in Infertility* (1975).

❦ *APPENDIX E*
Centers Offering New Conceptions

The following is a list of centers across the country offering services relating to the New Conceptions. This list is for informational purposes only and is not meant to serve as a recommendation for the programs listed. To learn of new facilities opening in your area or of additional practitioners offering the New Conceptions, contact the American Fertility Society, the American College of Obstetricians and Gynecologists, your state or local medical society, or the nearest large medical center.

IN VITRO FERTILIZATION PROGRAMS

- ### *CALIFORNIA*

Arnold Jacobson, M.D
John Muir Memorial Hospital
1601 Ygnacio Valley Rd.
Walnut Creek, CA 94598

William G. Karow, M.D.
California Institute for *In Vitro* Fertilization
12301 Wilshire Blvd., Suite 415
West Los Angeles, CA 90025

Richard Marrs, M.D. & Joyce Vargyas, M.D.
Univ. of Southern California - Women's Hospital of Los Angeles County
Department of Ob-Gyn
1240 N. Mission Road
Los Angeles, CA 90033

- ### *CONNECTICUT*

Alan De Cherney, M.D.
Yale University Medical School - Department of Ob-Gyn
333 Cedar St.
New Haven, CT 06510

Daniel H. Riddick, M.D.
Univ. of Conn. Health Center - John N. Dempsey Hospital
Div. of Reprod. Endocrinology & Infertility
Farmington, CT 06032

• *COLORADO*

George Henry, M.D.
Reproductive Genetics Center
St. Luke's Hospital
601 E. 19th Ave.
Denver, CO 80203

• *FLORIDA*

T. Hung, M.D.
University of Miami
Dept. of Ob-Gyn
P.O. Box 016960
Miami, FL 33101

• *GEORGIA*

Amir Ansari, M.D.
Georgia Baptist Medical Center - Department of Ob-Gyn
300 Boulevard N.E.
Atlanta, GA 30312

• *ILLINOIS*

Paul Dmowski, M.D.
Women's Health Consultants
1725 W. Harrison, Room 405
Chicago, IL 60612

Norbert Gleicher, M.D. & Jan Friberg, M.D.
Mount Sinai Hospital - Department of Ob-Gyn
California Avenue & 15th St.
Chicago, IL 60608

Antonio Scommegna, M.D.
Michael Reese Hospital - Department of Ob-Gyn
31st St. at Lake Shore Drive
Chicago, IL 60616

• *KANSAS*

Kermit Krantz
Univ. of Kansas College of Health Sciences
Bell Memorial Hospital
39th St. and Rainbow Blvd.
Kansas City, KS 66103

• *LOUISIANA*

Richard Dickey, M.D.
Pendleton Memorial Methodist Hospital
5620 Read Blvd.
New Orleans, LA 70127

• *MARYLAND*

John L. Young, M.D.
Genetic Consultants, Inc.
5616 Shields Drive
Bethesda, MD 20817

Theodore Baramski, M.D.
Greater Baltimore Medical Center
6701 N. Charles St.
Baltimore, MD 21204

John A. Rock, M.D.
Johns Hopkins Hospital - Div. of Reproductive Endocrinology
600 N. Wolfe St.
Baltimore, MD 21205

Union Memorial Hospital
East University Parkway
Baltimore, MD 21218

• *MASSACHUSETTS*

Beth Israel Hospital
330 Brookline Avenue
Boston, MA 02215

Brigham & Women's Hospital
75 Francis St.
Boston, MA 02115

- *MINNESOTA*

George Tagatz, M.D.
Univ. of Minn. Medical School - Ob-Gyn Dept.',
    Div. of Reprod. Endocrinology
Box 395, Mayo Memorial Building
Minneapolis, MN 55455

- *NEVADA*

Geoffrey Sher, M.D.
Reno Women's Clinic
350 W. 6th St.
Reno, NV 89503

- *NEW JERSEY*

Daniel W. Colburn, M.D. & Eckehard Kemman, M.D.
Middlesex General Hospital
180 Somerset St.
New Brunswick, NJ 08901

- *NEW YORK*

Raymond L. Vande Wiele, M.D. & Georgianna Jagiello, M.D.
Columbia Presbyterian Hospital Ob-Gyn Services
622 W. 168th St.
New York, NY 10032

Univ. of Rochester Medical Center
Department of Ob-Gyn
Rochester, NY 14627

CARE (Childbearing by Alternative Reproduction)
Strong Memorial Hospital of the University of Rochester
601 Elmwood Ave.
Rochester, NY 14642

- *NORTH CAROLINA*

Gary S. Berger, M.D.
Chapel Hill Fertility Services
109 Connor Drive, Suite 2104
Chapel Hill, NC 27514

Luther Talbert, M.D.
North Carolina Memorial Hospital
Dept. of Gynecology-Fertility Clinic
Chapel Hill, NC 27514

• *OHIO*

Ohio State University of Columbus
370 West 9th Avenue
Columbus, OH 43210

• *OKLAHOMA*

J. Clark Bundren, M.D. & J. W. Edward Wortham, M.D.
Hillcrest Infertility Center
1120 S. Utica
Tulsa, OK 74104

• *OREGON*

Oregon Health Sciences University
3181 S.W. Sam Jackson Park Blvd.
Portland, OR 97201

• *PENNSYLVANIA*

Luigi Mastroianni, M.D.
Presbyterian Univ. of Penn. Medical Center
51 North 39th St.
Philadelphia, PA 19104

Paul Zarutskie, M.D.
Magee - Women's Hospital
Forbes Ave. and Halket St.
Pittsburgh, PA 15213

• *TENNESSEE*

Anne Colston Wentz, M.D.
Vanderbilt University Medical Center
Center for Fertility and Reproductive Research
T-2302 Medical Center North
Nashville, TN 37232

• *TEXAS*

Raymond Kaufman, M.D.
Baylor College of Medicine - Department of Ob-Gyn
1200 Moursand Avenue
Houston, TX 77030

Martin M. Quigley, M.D.
Univ. of Texas Health Sciences Center - Reproductive Medicine Dept.
6431 Fannin, Suite 3270
Houston, TX 77030

Andrew Silverman, M.D. & Ricardo Asch, M.D.
Univ. of Texas Health Sciences Center - San Antonio - Dept. of Ob-Gyn
7703 Floyd Curl Drive
San Antonio, TX 78284

• *UTAH*

Richard Urry, M.D. and Richard Worley, M.D.
University of Utah *In Vitro* Clinic
University of Utah Hospital
50 N. Medical Dr.
Salt Lake City, UT 84132

• *VIRGINIA*

Howard W. Jones, Jr., M.D.
Eastern Virginia Medical School - Department of Ob-Gyn
600 Gresham Drive
Norfolk, VA 23507

• *WASHINGTON*

Laurence Karp, M.D.
Reproductive Genetics Group of the Division of Perinatal Medicine
Swedish Hospital Medical Center
747 Summit
Seattle, WA 98104

Michael Soules, M.D.
University Hospital
1959 N.E. Pacific St.
Seattle, WA 98195

• *WISCONSIN*

Univ. of Wisconsin Medical School - Infertility Clinic
1300 University Avenue
Madison, WI 53706

EMBRYO TRANSFER PROGRAMS

John Buster, M.D.
Harbor UCLA Medical Center
1000 W. Carson St.
Torrence, CA 90509

Randolph Seed, M.D. and Richard Seed, Ph.D.
The Reproduction & Fertility Clinic, Inc.
Water Tower Place
845 N. Michigan Ave.
Chicago, IL 60611

SURROGATE MOTHER PROGRAMS

William Handel
Sherwyn and Handel
8447 Wilshire Blvd.
Suite 301
Beverly Hills, CA 90211

Beth Bridgman, LMSW
The Hagar Institute
1808 Munson
Topeka, KS 66604

Katie Brophy
Surrogate Family Services Inc.
125 S. Seventh St.
Louisville, KY 40202

Richard Levin, M.D.
Surrogate Parenting Associates
Suite 222
Doctors' Office Building
250 East Liberty St.
Louisville, KY 40202

Harriet Blankfield
National Center for Surrogate Parenting
5530 Wisconsin Avenue
Chevy Chase, MD 20815

Noel Keane
930 Mason
Dearborn, MI 48124

Annette Ames
Ames Center for Surrogate Parenting, Inc.
P. O. Box 9201
Livonia, MI 48150

Kathryn Wyckoff
Association for Surrogate Parenting Services Inc.
4710 Chanterwood Dr.
Columbus, OH 43229

Burton Satzberg
Surrogate Mothering Limited
42 S. 15th
Philadelphia, PA 19102

❦ INDEX

Surrogate parenting *(cont.)*
  and contracts, 231, 233–236
  cost of, 203, 204, 206, 225, 252
  emotional aspects of, 199–201, 203,
    221, 268
  legal aspects of, 222, 226–233, 236,
    237–241
  medical aspects of, 201–202
  proposed legislation for, 237–241
  readings on, 302–305
  social aspects of, 223–225
Surrogate parenting centers, 205–207,
    210–211, 216, 218, 220, 231, 232,
    235, 317–318

Tay-Sachs disease and trait, 61, 68,
    71–72, 168, 169–170
Test-tube babies. *See In vitro
    fertilization*
Testicle(s)
  biopsy of, 51, 109, 163–164
  examination of, 49
  transplant, 244
Testosterone, for low sperm counts, 53
Thalessemia, 61
Transcervical aspiration, 66
Transcutaneous needle aspiration, in
    egg retrieval, 131
Transfer of donor oocytes. *See Egg do-
    nation*
Transplants
  of fallopian tube, 244
  of ovary, 244
  of testicle, 244

Treatment technologies, and infertility,
    23–25
Tubal cautery, 28, 123
Tubal ligation, 27
  reversal of, 27–28
Tubal occlusion, bilateral, 28
Tubal problems
  evaluation of, 40–43
  IVF for, 122–123, 199
  surrogate mothering for, 198
Tuboplasty, 48
Turner's syndrome, 68, 69

Ultrasound
  in genetic screening, 65, 66, 77
  in IVF, 129, 131

Varicocele, 49–50, 53, 123
  AID in, 163
Vasectomy, 27
  reversal of, 28–29, 53
Vasogram, 51
Veneral disease
  and infertility, 29
  screening sperm donors for, 167–168

Woman, single, AID for, 192, 193–195
Workplace hazards, and infertility, 10,
    22–23

X, Fragile, 61–62
X-Linked disorders, 61–62, 88
XYY syndrome, 84